clean cures

the humble art of zen-curing yourself

by michael dejong

a joost elffers production

STERLING

New York / London
www.sterlingpublishing.com

STERLING and the distinctive Sterling logo are registered trademarks of Sterling Publishing Co., Inc.

10 9 8 7 6 5 4 3 2 1

Published by Sterling Publishing Co., Inc.
387 Park Avenue South, New York, NY 10016

This book is printed in a sustainable manner using 100 percent (post- and pre-consumer) recycled paper and vegetable-based inks. No new trees were used.

CLEAN CURES
The Humble Art of Zen-Curing Yourself
A Joost Elffers Production

Distributed in Canada by Sterling Publishing
c/o Canadian Manda Group, 165 Dufferin Street
Toronto, Ontario, Canada M6K 3H6
Distributed in the United Kingdom by GMC Distribution Services
Castle Place, 166 High Street, Lewes, East Sussex, England BN7 1XU
Distributed in Australia by Capricorn Link (Australia) Pty. Ltd.
P.O. Box 704, Windsor, NSW 2756, Australia

Design and illustration by Yumi Asai and Edgar Prieto at Berrymatch LLC

Printed in China

Sterling ISBN 978-1-4027-6697-8

For information about custom editions, special sales, premium and corporate purchases, please contact Sterling Special Sales Department at 800-805-5489 or specialsales@sterlingpublishing.com.

To my partner, Richard Haymes ~
Who's just what the doctor ordered.

ACKNOWLEDGMENTS

"Clean Cures" wouldn't have been possible without the first aid of the following people:

Teresa Heinz for encouraging my written treatments.

Lindy Judge for her infectious, tender loving care.

Yumi Asai for her blistering attention to detail.

Michael Fragnito for promoting this operation.

Barbara Berger for suturing it all together.

Jenny Clad for her dose of good humor.

Dr. Vavasis for examining my content.

Joost Elffers for his feverish insight.

FOREWORD

As a family doctor, I have always tried to give my patients treatments that will help them to feel better while exposing them to the least harm. Over the years, I have tried to add to my treatment repertoire as many ideas that begin with the words "My grandmother always recommended..." as possible. In this spirit, Michael DeJong has done extensive research to identify simple, safe treatments for common medical problems that would make our collective grandmother proud. While this book does not eliminate the need for my profession entirely, I hope that it will give you a few ideas of how to use six simple ingredients to relieve common problems. Leave the serious or chronic medical problems to your medical provider, but for the more minor ones, use *Clean Cures* to heal thyself.

Anthony Vavasis, M.D.

Index

	apple cider vinegar	baking soda	honey	lemon	olive oil	salt	pages
D							
Dandruff	x	x	x		x	x	85
Dermatitis	x	x			x	x	86
Diarrhea	x	x	x	x			87
Digestion	x		x	x	x		88
Dry Mouth		x	x	x		x	89
E							
Earache	x				x	x	91
Eczema	x	x	x		x	x	92
Eyes, Dry	x	x	x	x		x	93
F							
Fatigue	x		x	x		x	95
Fever	x	x	x	x			96
Fever Blisters	x	x	x	x	x	x	75, 97
Flatulence	x	x		x	x		99
Flea Bites	x	x		x			100

	apple cider vinegar	baking soda	honey	lemon	olive oil	salt	pages
Heat Rash	x	x		x	x		115
Hemorrhoids	x	x	x	x	x		116
Hiccups	x	x	x	x		x	118
Hives	x	x			x	x	119
Hoarseness	x		x	x		x	120, 133
Hot Flashes	x	x	x	x	x		120
Hyperactivity	x		x				121
I							
Indigestion	x	x	x	x			123
Inflammation	x		x				124, 174
Ingrown Hair	x	x	x			x	124
Ingrown Toenails	x			x	x	x	125
Insect Stings & Bites	x	x	x	x	x	x	126
Insomnia	x	x	x	x	x	x	128
Itchy Skin	x	x	x		x	x	92, 130

	apple cider vinegar	baking soda	honey	lemon	olive oil	salt	pages
R							
Rashes	x	x	x	x	x	x	155
Razor Burn	x	x	x		x		156
S							
Sinus Headache	x	x		x		x	159
Sneezing	x	x	x	x		x	160
Snoring	x		x		x	x	162
Sore Gums	x	x	x	x		x	163
Sore Throat	x	x	x	x		x	164
Splinters	x		x	x	x	x	84, 165
Sprains	x				x		165
Stiff Neck	x			x	x		166
Stiffness	x	x	x	x	x	x	167
Stings & Bites, Insect	x	x	x	x	x	x	126, 167
Stomachache	x	x	x				168
Stomach, Upset	x	x	x	x			123, 168
Stress	x	x	x		x		169

	apple cider vinegar	baking soda	honey	lemon	olive oil	salt	pages
Windburn	x	x		x	x		183
Wounds & Cuts	x		x	x	x	x	184
Wrinkles	x	x	x	x	x		186
Y							
Yeast Infection	x	x				x	189

INTRODUCTION

"Words of kindness are more healing to a drooping heart than balm or honey."
~ SARAH FIELDING

I'm a pretty healthy guy…some might say fit as a fiddle. But, on an off day here and there, when I'm under the weather, it's no day at the park—for me or for anyone who has to put up with me. I've also been around folks who aren't feeling up to snuff as well. You know who they are—adults with hangovers, preteens with pimples, gardeners with blisters, beauty queens with chapped lips, newborns with cradle cap, construction workers with headaches, kids with head lice, hikers with heat exhaustion, campers with insect bites, students with insomnia, vacationers with jet lag, weekend warriors with muscle aches, beachcombers with sunburn, or just the common Joe or Jane with a stuffy nose.

The importance of wellness is obvious - there's nothing like feeling swell. If you don't feel good you're not going to be functioning at your finest.

Through the course of your day—between waking and sleeping—you might get a bump or a scratch, catch a bug or simply overdo it. From slight to excruciating—above par, so-so, or under-the-covers needing to be alone—depending on who you are, the effects of your ailments will differ greatly from how they might affect others with the same ones. And although nobody likes it, the suffering that goes along with not feeling great is part of our shared human condition.

Throughout history, poor health, discomfort, and suffering have played important roles in many religions. For instance, Buddhists consider the release from illness and suffering basic to any holy life, Hindus believe that infirmity is the consequence of unfortunate past behavior, and the Bible's Book of Job also discusses the metaphor of sickness.

Many Eastern traditions posit that the universe is controlled by the dance of the elements. When combined with the duality of Yin and Yang, these elemental mixtures generate contrast, tension, conflict, and balance. Much like the Buddhist six elements of Earth, Water, Fire, Air, Space, and Consciousness, the six essentials in *Clean Cures* perform similarly with chains of reaction and interaction, blending and balancing for a mindful, integrated healing experience.

The six pure and simple elements used in *Clean Cures* are:

Apple Cider Vinegar
Baking Soda
Honey
Lemon
Olive Oil
Salt

Not newfangled or exotic, each of the six ingredients has its own time-honored qualities—alone or in unison—to comfort and heal. Safely used for millenium, you probably have many of them in your pantry. So, while "new and improved" expensive commercial remedies continue to pile high on drugstore shelves, humble apple cider vinegar, baking soda, honey, lemon, olive oil, and salt are not "new" and need no "improving"—they have already proven themselves to be steadfast, scrumptious and safe.

In addition to the six common ingredients, *Clean Cures*' basics require only a few every-day items to administer them effectively—measuring cups, eight-ounce drinking glasses, teaspoons and tablespoons, recycled covered glass or plastic jars, an eye dropper, an ear syringe, clean cotton cloths or towels, white cotton socks, and some sterile gauze and bandages are probably all you need to have on hand.

Packaging (or should I say over-packaging) from commercially prepared over-the-counter capsules, creams, preparations, syrups, and tonics always get tossed into the trash. (And am I the only one who finds it impossible to open those single pill blister packets?) *Clean Cures* remedies eliminate the need to purchase those pre-packaged, often petrochemical-related products in the first place. Imagine all of the plastic, paper, foil, cardboard, cotton, and glass that will no longer need to be manufactured, recycled or end up in landfills across the country. It might seem trivial, but multiplied by millions of homes our joined effort can have a huge effect.

For instance, take a very simple thing like a tube of lip balm, with casings made from plastic, each on average measuring about 2½ inches in length and weighing just about .15 ounces when full. Keeping in mind that the average person goes through about four per year—in the US alone—discarded and lined up end to end, they'd stretch nearly 2½ round-trips to the moon and weigh as much as 1,838 Liberty Bells! And to top it all off, lip balm plastic casings have no indication on them that they are suitable for recycling.

So you can see that *Clean Cures* isn't just about wellness. In an attempt to reclaim our environment, and save our planet, it's also an alternative to mass consumerism and an avenue to mass participation. *Clean Cures* offers but one small way in which we can not only heal minor ailments naturally and effectively, but also a way to protect our cherished relations, our acquaintances, our adored pets, ourselves and our ailing Mother Earth.

Though standard health care does its very best to address the suffering often affiliated with illness, there are many ways to relieve minor aches and pains with simple treatments—tried-and-true old-as-the-hills alternatives that our grandparents and probably their grandparents and their grandparents used. Some of these remedies go back as far as the ancient Egyptians, Greeks, and Romans. And before the advent of modern chemical laboratory-produced first aid treatments, some were still being successfully used during World War I.

So whether you're an eco-freak, a person overly concerned about his or her health, or just someone sick and tired of medicating every ache, sniffle, or sneeze with ointments for infections, powders for pain, salves for scrapes, or balms for bites, *Clean Cures* is chock-a-block with affordable, healthful, thoughtful alternatives for many common minor ailments.

In Zen, we're all the product of our intentions—every action, no matter how small, makes a difference. If you're sick, your world is sick. When you're healthy, so is your life. Each moment—healthy or ill—makes a difference because each one leads to the next. In an attempt to safeguard our precious health, we need to carefully nurture and develop our ability to mindfully care for ourselves. A daily "dose of mindfulness" can lead to an eco-effective existence. In the words of the ancient Roman philosopher, Virgil, *"The greatest wealth is health."*

So whether you're anyone from a mother to-be with morning sickness to a traveler with motion sickness, *Clean Cures* can help you naturally preserve or restore your state of well-being by showing you how to carefully take care.

PREFACE

"There's a remedy for all things but death."

~MIGUEL DE CERVANTES

I'm not a fan of going to the doctor, and I'll sniffle and cough for up to a week before I'll actually take an over-the-counter medication. Instead, I'll sip steaming apple cider vinegar; drink lemony hot liquids and belly up to what my partner Richard likes to call Jewish penicillin (a crock-pot of homemade chicken soup), all while cleaning the house out of frustration and boredom in an attempt to relieve and comfort myself.

When I have a cold, despite the fact that I'm sneezing or coughing, I'll still vacuum almost daily, albeit in my nightshirt, while wiping my runny nose on the tissues that Richard keeps within reach from any location in the house. I'll sleep as much as I can, mindlessly absorb hours of unseen episodes of *CSI* (the Las Vegas edition with Marg Helgenberger, only! I might not feel my best, but I do try to maintain my standards.), take comforting hot baths, and soothe myself with balms and steam until the worst of the worst is over. As my partner likes to tell me, "the cold is going to take seven days to a week to get over—whichever comes first." And not being a person who can sit still for very long, when I'm down for the old "one-two" punch of a cold or some other nonthreatening ailment...man-oh-man, am I crabby! (Besides being irritable, I want relief...NOW, NOW, NOW!) At over six feet, I'm a big guy, but when I feel crummy, I might as well be a toddler in tears. (Hey, I'm allowed to be difficult...I'm sick!)

But over the years, I've learned that there are things I can do to help myself (and thus help those who have to be around me when I'm under the weather). Having the necessary raw ingredients—apple cider vinegar, baking soda, honey, lemon, olive oil and/or salt—to speed me along the road to wellness eliminates my necessity to get dressed, bundle up, deal with the elements, and walk or drive to the drugstore only to elbow the hordes of other sick, snarky, short-tempered folks who are attempting in glassy-eyed befuddlement to read—let alone understand—the labels of the countless and expensive over-the-counter medications lining shelf after shelf. Lately, whenever I've been in that moment of thinking I need to run out to the pharmacy, I've stopped and said to myself, "Michael, the best remedy for ill-health is good-health, and even poor-health is sometimes easier on me than the side-effects of those so-called 'cures.'" And then I take my own advice and follow the recipes I've compiled in this book.

With the medical industry placing a cost on everything—insurance premiums (if you're lucky enough to be in a plan), pharmaceuticals, lab tests, co-pays, etc.—nobody wants, and few of us can afford, to put a price tag on our own health. But pricey it is, and even over-the-counter medications can be costly. The remedies in this book, however, are super cheap! And they're also made from natural, safe ingredients, have no negative side effects, are chemical free, and have been around for millennia (long before the age of mass-marketed treatments and televised promotion of pharmaceuticals. You know, the ads where a very fast talker rattles off all the potential side effects—headaches, heart palpitations, rashes, anal leakage anyone!?—at the very end of the slickly produced commercial).

Nature can be a wonderful healer, and there are plenty of time-honored home remedies for your aches and pains, blisters and bunions that can be made from items found as close by as your pantry or fridge.

The myriad of modern over-the-counter drugs we now take for granted—cough suppressants and expectorants, decongestants, headache relievers, solutions for constipation, mole treatments, fungal preparations, and antibiotic ointments for wounds—didn't always exist. Not to say that these nonprescription medications don't offer relief (they often do because they mask the symptoms) but, truth be told, most have side effects worse than the actual aliment.

Don't get me wrong. There are heaps of commercial concoctions, brews and tonics to comfort, calm, ease and soothe you in your moment of need—many of which work well, are in harmony with the environment, and are safe for consumption—though you probably won't find them in big box stores or chain pharmacies. But you don't need to pay the high cost of commercial concoctions or surf the Internet to locate some remote retailer of the green and clean remedies you desire. You can safely make them yourself, right at home.

What I've compiled here in *Clean Cures* is a collection of interesting and useful healthcare tips to offer a ship of calm in a stormy sea. Although I've assembled the following home remedies and natural treatments, please keep in mind that I am not a doctor or any other kind of medical expert (nor have I ever played one on TV!). The details and remedies included here aim at being educational and informative, and aren't intended to substitute for qualified medical advice, a comprehensive medical exam, or the TLC offered by those in the health care profession. Always speak to your doctor or pharmacist before taking any prescriptions, over-the-counter medications or even the home remedies in this book. Only your doctor or pharmacist can supply the specific kind of guidance that's beneficial, safe, and effective for you.

And always bear in mind that being under the weather is one thing, but if you find yourself seriously ill, definitely visit a medical practitioner, call 911, or get to an emergency room. These remedies are not intended to replace current prescriptions you may be on for serious acute or chronic illnesses. Always check with your pharmacist or health care provider to make sure none of the ingredients in the remedies in this book would interfere with or be contraindicative with any medications you might be taking. However, while waiting to see your health care provider for minor things that ail you, consider trying these natural and safe treatments at home.

Aching muscles, acne, age spots, or allergies—with some simple knowledge and a grasp of the power of natural remedies you can forgo the strong chemicals normally used to treat a range of nonthreatening conditions. And since prescription medications (everything from female replacement hormones to Viagra) have recently been found in microscopic portions in ordinary drinking water, at least you can rest assured that the ingredients in these home remedies are eco-friendly and will not further pollute our planet—or your body.

THE INGREDIENTS

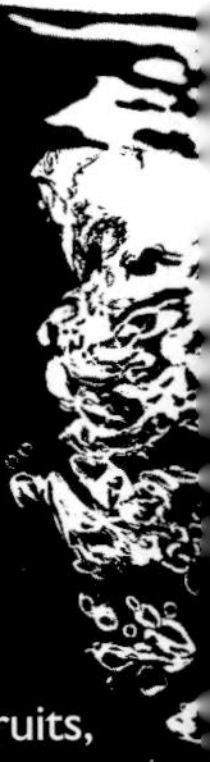

APPLE CIDER VINEGAR

Vinegar, from the French for "sour wine," is produced from assorted fruits, berries, melons, coconut, honey, beer, maple syrup, potatoes, beets, malt, grains, and whey. But no matter what the original ingredient may be, the production in essence remains unaltered: a first fermentation of sugar to alcohol, then a second fermentation to vinegar. Simply put: Fermented fruit? Voilà...Vinegar! Acetic acid is born.

Sharp, sour, and biting, the smack of vinegar, to most of us, always remains the same. But the flavor definitely differs from one to another. There's wine vinegar, rice vinegar, apple cider vinegar, tarragon vinegar, balsamic vinegar, and any number of other exotic blends.

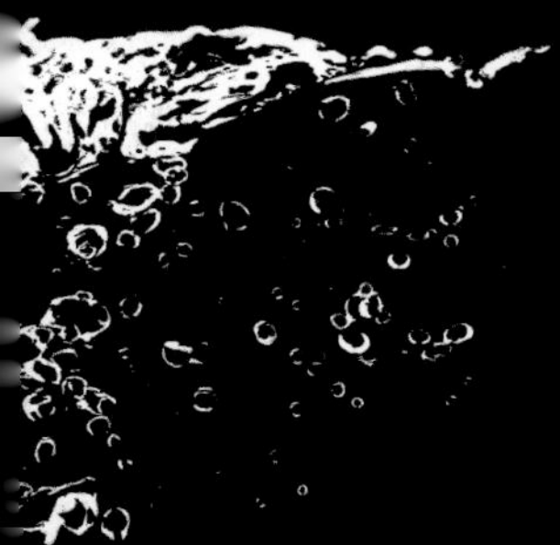

But for the purposes of *Clean Cures*, I'm talking about that familiar, yet forgotten, bottle of "apple cider vinegar" that's probably lurking in your pantry hidden behind the cans of pinto beans, jars of pickles, stacks of cookie sheets, and cookbooks.

Apple cider vinegar is a type of vinegar made by fermenting apple cider. The sugar in the apple cider is broken down by bacteria and yeast into alcohol and then again into vinegar. It contains acetic acid (like other types of vinegar) along with some lactic, citric, and malic acids.

Unlike distilled white vinegar, which was an ingredient in *Clean: The Humble Art of Zen-Cleansing* and *Clean Body: The Humble Art of Zen-Cleansing Yourself,*

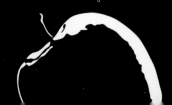

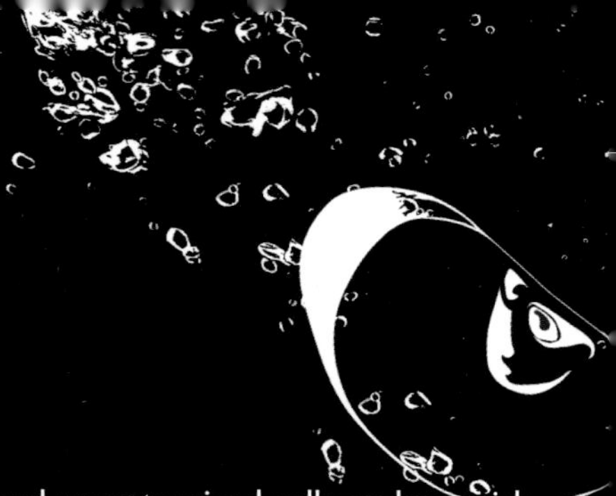

apple cider vinegar is the unfiltered and unpasteurized yellowy-brownish stepsister. Sold in health food stores, online, and in some grocery stores, apple cider vinegar often contains a dark, cloudy sediment called "mother of vinegar" that has settled at the bottom of the bottle.

Other types of vinegar—such as white vinegar, balsamic vinegar, red wine vinegar, and rice wine vinegar—can be used for both cooking and cleaning. Apple cider vinegar, however, is best used for health purposes.

This multipurpose elixir can linger eternally, refrigerated or not, making it easy to store and use. Given a good dusting, that bottle of pungent, piquant liquid is versatile both gastronomically and medicinally.

The ancients stumbled upon the versatility of vinegar probably 10,000 years ago. The Babylonians used it as medicine and flavored their meals with vinegar and herbs. Hippocrates consumed apple cider vinegar as a health tonic. The Romans drank it as a beverage. Cleopatra dissolved pearls in it to prove she could devour a fortune in a single meal. Biblical references show how it was used for its soothing and healing properties, and as recently as World War I, vinegar was still being used to treat wounds in the battlefields.

It's said, "You catch more flies with honey than you do with vinegar," implying the virtues of sweetness over bitterness. But in the case of *Clean Cures*, it is precisely the acidic virtues of apple cider vinegar that make it such a sweet, soothing treasure. Store plenty in a tightly sealed container and keep it close at hand because many *Clean Cures* recipes rely on this deliciously "bitter" potion.

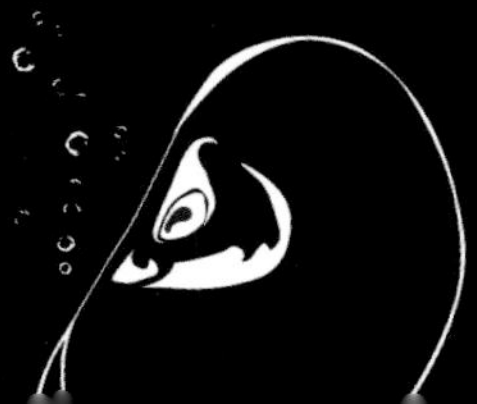

BAKING SODA

Fresh from its familiar, iconic carton, the white, soft and dusty-dry gems of baking soda shimmer like Caribbean sands. That ubiquitous open box of baking soda, obscured behind the onions and oranges, anchovies and apples, works silently and magically, absorbing all sorts of odors. But baking soda can do a lot more than just mask the malodorous.

Our forefathers produced primitive baking sodas and gave them wonderful names like *saleratus*, *trona,* or *nitre*. American frontiersmen fashioned a version of it from the cinders of scorched corn, and transformed it into any number of practical (as well as "snake-oil") purposes, such as cure-alls for asthma, powders for cleanliness, balms for baldness, and treatments for dry and chapped skin.

Hygiene and health with baking soda, however, goes back a lot further than the Wild, Wild West—all the way back to Biblical times. "For though thou wash with nitre, and take thee much soap, yet thine iniquity is marked before me, saith the Lord God" (Jeremiah 2:22). In ancient Egypt, when used to mummify the remains of great Pharaohs, not only did baking soda clean the body, it preserved it as well.

Established in the beds of Egyptian lakes, the crystals form when water in the heated desert climate evaporates. Traded for thousands of years, Egyptian writings as old as the reign of Ramses III refer to these deposits.

Sprinkled, scattered, spread or strewn, kept in your closet, kitty litter, salad crisper, or carport—baking soda in any of its namesakes is powerful enough to preserve the dead. (Not a "Do It Yourself" project! Kids, do not try this at home!) But today, its strength can be used not only to sweeten, clean, and freshen your home, but also to relieve an upset tummy, cure acne, prevent smelly feet and BO, make a relaxing and healing bath, and even serve as a soothing eyewash. Baking soda will be one of the most effective, most versatile, and most often-used ingredients in the *Clean Cures* family of six basic elements.

HONEY

Conjuring an everlasting image of sweetness, distinctively golden yellow, viscous, gooey, and sticky, honey is the delicious saccharine yet syrupy by-product from honeybees collecting nectar while pollinating.

Depending on where the bees buzz, honey can be enriched with either the flavors of alfalfa, blackberry, buckwheat, clover, dandelion, eucalyptus, goldenrod, orange blossom, sage, or sourwood. Primarily used in cooking, baking, as a quick and yummy topping on toast, or simply to sweeten beverages, throughout history honey has also had symbolic meaning.

In the Jewish tradition, for example, apple slices are dipped in honey to symbolize sweetness for the New Year. In Buddhist culture, it was once brought to Buddha as a gift. The phrase "land flowing with milk and honey" is a Biblical description of Israel. Aristotle wrote of using the syrupy stuff as

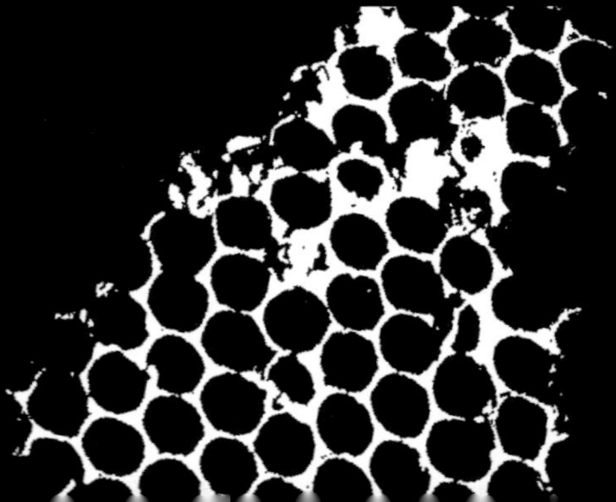

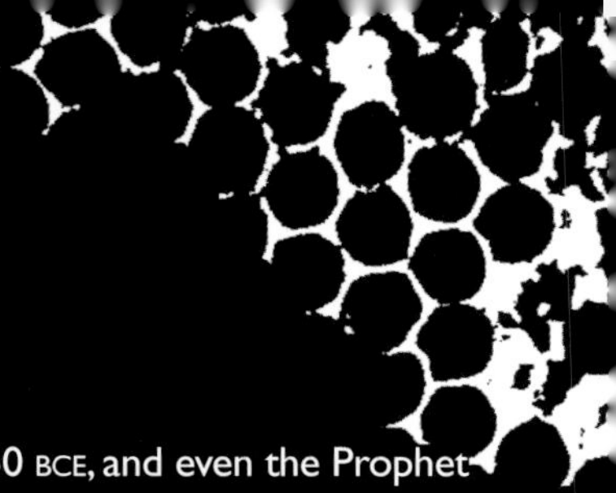

an unguent for sores and abrasions around 350 BCE, and even the Prophet Muhammad recommended honey for healing. Surprisingly antiseptic and antibacterial simultaneously, it's also perfect for aliments from sore throats to sore tummies.

Produced in most countries of the world, crystallized, heat-treated, organic, raw, strained, ultra-filtered, in a bear-shaped jar, or still on the comb, honey is the sweetest of the six *Clean Cures* ingredients. But as the Chinese proverb says "Sour, sweet, bitter, pungent, all must be tasted."

One of the finest foods we can store for survival, honey—kept under proper conditions—can last indefinitely.

(Note of Caution: *Honey can be dangerous to infants under the age of one.*)

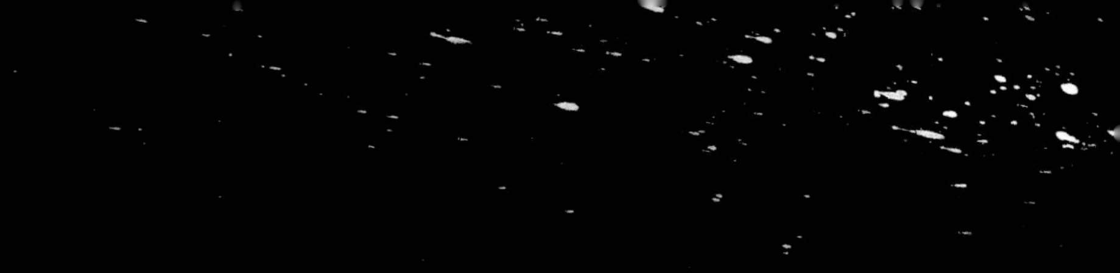

LEMON

Strong, sharp, acidic, and citrus-sassy, the light golden lemon offers sun-ripened effervescence—either picked ripe from the tree or found in the produce section of your supermarket. With sharp thorns and twigs, oblong leaves, and fragrant buds of reddish hues that bloom into white and lavender flowers, the lemon fruit is light yellow, oval, and aromatic. Dotted with oil glands that produce its memorable scent and hidden beneath a sun-ripened tough exterior of rind lies its acidic juicy segments. For some, just the thought of a lemon can make their mouths water, for others even the notion of all that tartness makes their mouths pucker up.

Lemons aren't just for fish and tea anymore, as you'll soon see! The eight to ten perfect sections protected under a leathery exterior offer up what was once prized by sultans, gifted by kings and traded across the conti-

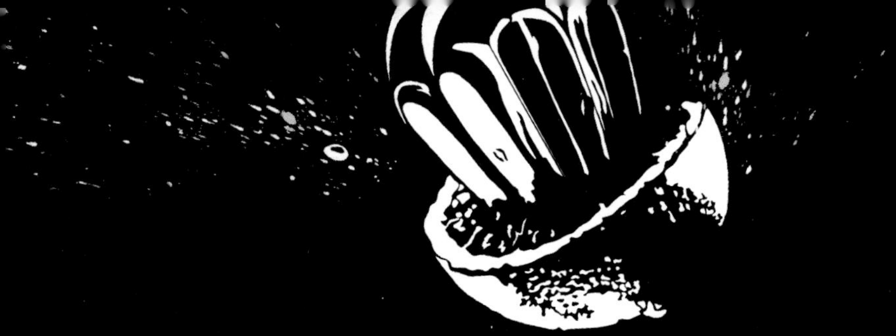

nents by sailors, pirates, and smugglers. Although its origin is unknown, the lemon is believed to have been cultivated in ancient Iraq and Egypt. It is also rumored that Christopher Columbus carried its seeds in his vest pockets. Today the tart and succulent fruit is grown in Italy, Spain, Greece, Turkey, Cyprus, Lebanon, South Africa, Australia and the Philippines, as well as in the United States.

Not all that long ago, the now humble lemon was highly coveted by adventurous seafarers and pillaged by plunderers. In the process, the vitamin-C-rich fruit made its way from continent to continent, carried by explorers, bandits, and outcasts. In fact, on his very first voyage to the South Pacific, from Fiji to Samoa and Tahiti to Tonga, Captain Cook mysteriously lost half of his crew to illness. Once it was determined that the cause was scurvy, the significance of consuming citrus for vitamin C while at sea was established. (Hence, the term "Limeys" for English sailors.) Nowadays most of us get our "C" from a balanced diet or by taking supplements.

With names like Armstrong, Bearss, Berna, Eureka, Femminello Ovale, Genoa, Harvey, Interdonato, Lisbon, Meyer, Monachello, Nepali Oblong, Nepali Round, Perrine, Ponderosa, Rosenberger, Rough Lemon, Santa Teresa, Sweet Lemon, and Villafranca, the common lemon really isn't "oh-so-common" after all. Each variety varies slightly in color, texture, shape, flavor, and scent. And whether you choose the exotic or the mundane variety, any lemon you can get your hands on will certainly do the trick as a *Clean Cures* ingredient.

A bowl of a dozen placed casually out in the open, and another bunch tossed into your crisper or stashed in your refrigerator door, will make living with the most perishable of the six elements all the easier. But wherever you choose to keep them, keep plenty on hand as lemons are an essential ingredient in *Clean Cures*' home remedies. And let's not forget that they taste great on salads and make any room smell fresh and clean!

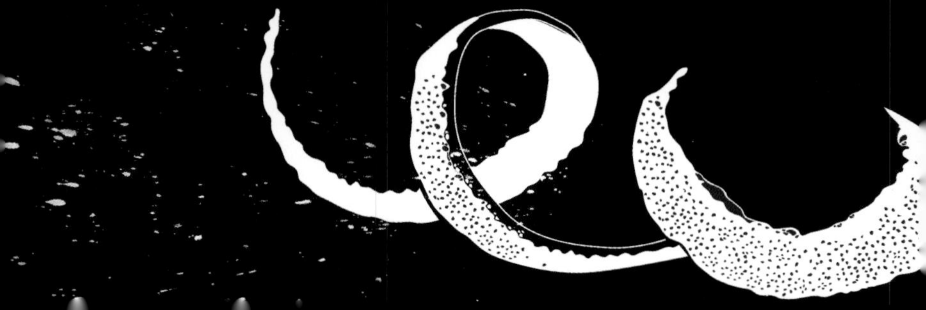

OLIVE OIL

Whether pale yellow, "olive green," or honey-amber; cold-pressed, virgin, or extra-virgin—olive oil is remarkably versatile and has long served as more than the main ingredient in the perfect vinaigrette. As you'll soon discover, this traditional, luxurious oil goes way beyond being just a fabulous food. And it requires no refrigeration, making it easy to store and use.

Available just about everywhere—from gourmet shops to the local bodega—olive oil is considered a basic household staple and has been used for a variety of nonfood purposes for centuries. Muhammad used its richness to anoint himself and the heads of his disciples, and it is often used for baptism ceremonies in Christianity. This yummy lubricant was also used to bless early rulers as well as winning athletes, and since Biblical times, the olive branch has been recognized as a universal symbol of peace.

Used in the burial process in ancient Egypt, it was believed that the fruit, branches, leaves, and oil of the olive tree, when included in the departed's sarcophagus, would ensure a safe and pleasant passage to the underworld by protecting the souls of the dead from evil spirits.

But olive oil's powers go beyond protecting the souls of the dead. In fact, olive oil is equally essential to the living, for whom it can help with rashes, reduce razor burn, be used as a wonderful massage lubricant, and help diminish stretch marks.

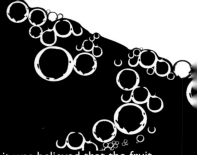

SALT

Lustrous, brilliantly white, and crystalline, salt is one of the most plentiful and useful minerals on earth. We enhance our culinary creations with it; melt icy sidewalks with it; and many cultures have even created parables about it. Planets in outer space are filled with gi-normous bubbling molten oceans of it, while here on Earth, we race cars on Great Plains of it, buoyantly swim in turquoise-colored oceans of it, and even "take the cure" in it. Stored in shakers displayed on dining tables or found next to stovetops in heaping bowls, the coarse, granular, or powdery pale element stands ready to offer the handy pinch to almost every sweet or savory culinary invention. And while you'll still shake it over your fries, now *Clean Cures* will have you using it in ways you never imagined!

Listed on the periodic table of elements, iodized, sea, bay, kosher, canning, pickling, or rock salt, sodium chloride occurs naturally in soil and water. Salt

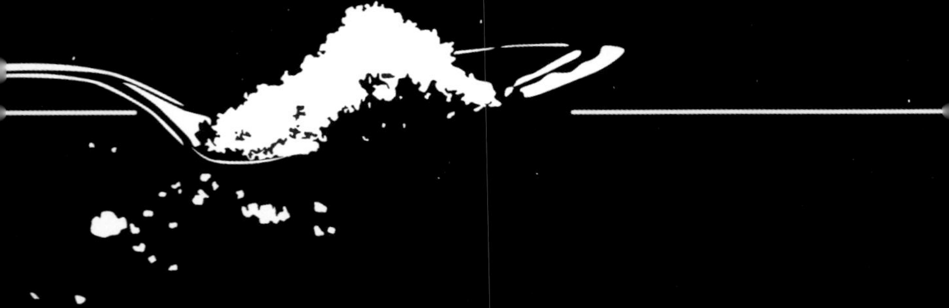

is the fourth most abundant element on earth. Like baking soda, it too was used to preserve the remains of the ancient Pharaohs.

Throughout the ages, salt has been extremely important to people and cultures. No less than thirty references to salt are made in the Bible. Lot's wife was transformed into a cold and bloodless pillar of the stuff when, even though she was warned not to, she just had to turn to see the fall of Gomorrah. Roman soldiers of antiquity were often paid in salt, and this was called their *salarium*, from which our word "salary" is derived. Once paid, the salt could be used as money in exchange for other goods. It was said that a good soldier was "worth his salt," a term still used for a worthy person.

Superstition has it that if spilled, you should toss some of it over your left shoulder to ward off bad luck. Not that I believe it, but. . .ya' know, it can't hurt. But don't waste too much of it—it's far too useful! Salt is indeed worth its weight—it's not just practical in the kitchen or for homemade housecleaning projects, or for its beauty applications. As you'll see, salt is an important ingredient in *Clean Cures*; it has extraordinary antiseptic qualities, works as a super sterilizer, and even serves as a dynamic disinfectant.

REMEDIES

DISCLAIMER: Please know that I'm not a doctor or a medical expert of any kind. The information contained in *Clean Cures* is intended as an educational aid for simple, alternative home remedies only. The remedies contained in this book are not intended as a replacement for professional medical advice or as a substitute for a health consultation for individual conditions or treatments. It is not a substitute for a medical exam, nor does it replace the need for services that can only be provided by licensed medical professionals. Before trying these or any other remedies, it is suggested that you speak with your doctor or pharmacist before following any treatment or regimen because only a medical professional can provide you with advice on what is safe and effective for you.

The following information is supplied for interest only and is not intended as a medical guide, nor is it comprehensive in any way. A growing number of people are now wishing to live a sustainable and eco-effective lifestyle, and this book is intended to illustrate that for some simple ailments there are some simple remedies made from simple ingredients. Any individual who chooses to use them, however, does so of his or her own free will and should always exercise common sense. Neither I nor my publisher will be held responsible for any negative side effects resulting from the use of these remedies. If you are sick, injured, or traumatized, rather than attempting to heal yourself with these home remedies, please visit a medical practitioner, or in the case of an emergency, call 911 immediately.

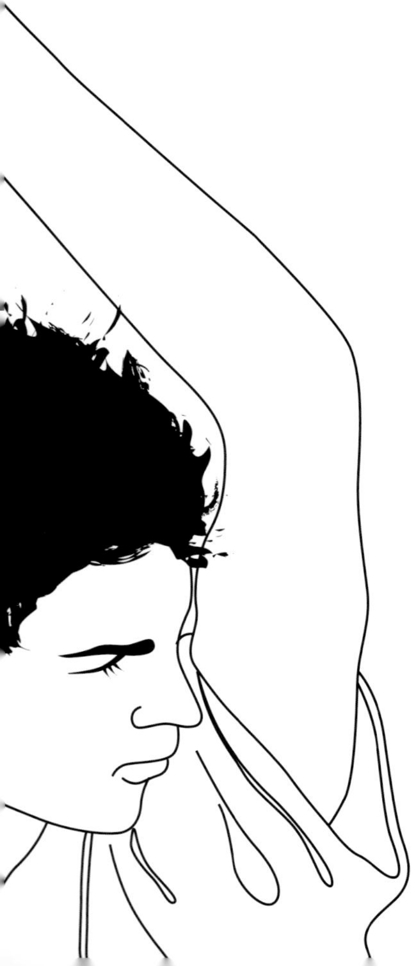

ACHING JOINTS

Aching joints are usually due to inflammation in the joints or degeneration of the cartilage where your bones are connected. As we age, we complain about our aching joints in our hands, knees, elbows, shoulders, and feet. While sometimes caused by overexertion, inflexible, swollen, or painful joints may be experienced by young and old.

Use your "smarts" and try the following to bring ease to your aching joints:

APPLE CIDER VINEGAR

- Soak a clean old towel in a mixture of ¼ cup of apple cider vinegar and 1½ cups of hot water. Wrap the painful area with the hot, wet towel, and cover with another dry cloth to trap in the heat. Remove when the wet towel gets cooler. Repeat several times for greater relief. Because apple cider vinegar may stain light fabrics, it's best to use old or darker colored towels for this remedy.

HONEY

- Lightly rub your painful joints with honey for ten minutes before bedtime and then wrap with a warm cloth overnight.

LEMON

- To relieve joint pains, shave off a slice of the yellow peel of a lemon and rub it gently onto aching areas releasing the lemon's oil. Then, hold the peel in place with a bandage and let it work its healing effect for an hour or two.

OLIVE OIL

- Eating at least one tablespoon of olive oil each day can improve your overall health. This serving can also act to improve your joint mobility.

SALT

- A cup of salt diluted in a warm bath may help to reduce your inflammation.

CAUTION: *If aching joints are the result of a trauma or if they are red and feel hot, you should be evaluated immediately by a medical professional.*

ACHING MUSCLES

Aching muscles are commonly caused by overstretching, overusing, and generally over doing it—especially if you're not used to it. Certain folks experience achy and sore muscles from physical strain often experienced as muscle fatigue and exhaustion.

The next time you do too much and feel the achy and painful aftermath, exercise some of these solutions:

APPLE CIDER VINEGAR

- To treat muscle aches and pains, soak in a tub full of warm water with two cups of apple cider vinegar added. Give it a stir and soak for thirty minutes.

BAKING SODA

- Soak in a warm bath with a half cup of baking soda for about thirty to sixty minutes.

OLIVE OIL

- Warm a tablespoon of olive oil and massage it into your aching muscles.

CAUTION: *If aching muscles are a result of trauma, you should be evaluated immediately by a medical professional.*

ACNE

Outbreaks make you face your acne.

When your pores get clogged and inflamed, you unfortunately end up with acne. The surface of your skin gets choked causing those icky blackheads and whiteheads we've all come to dread. Surprisingly, more adults get acne than teenagers. And if that's not bad enough, although we've all done it, squeezing or popping pimples causes pitting and scars…so don't!

For zapping your zits—just a pinch of this and that works best—and you'll also burst with joy when you use the following treatments:

APPLE CIDER VINEGAR

- To loosen dirt and oil, steam your face over a pan of boiling water while placing a towel over your head to trap the steam. Then apply apple cider vinegar with a cotton ball to remove the dirt and oil. Finish by dabbing more apple cider vinegar onto your pores to close them.

BAKING SODA

- To create an effective scrub, mix a tablespoon of baking soda with enough water to form a paste. Carefully apply it to your face and gently massage it into your skin for ten to fifteen seconds. Rinse your face completely with warm water and pat dry with a clean towel.

HONEY

- Apply honey onto your problem pimples after thoroughly cleansing your skin. Keep the honey on the affected area for about ten minutes, and then rinse off with warm water.

LEMON

- Wipe fresh lemon juice onto your pimples with a cotton ball or swab before bedtime. In the morning, you'll start your day with a fresh face.

SALT

- Sprinkle a teaspoon of salt into the palm of your hand and add just a bit of warm water until you make a paste. Rub the moistened mixture over your acne. Let it set for a minute, rinse your skin clean with warm water, and then gently pat dry with a clean towel.

CAUTION: *Whiteheads are clogged pores below the outer layer of your skin and should never be squeezed. Blackheads are clogged pores on the surface and also should not be scrubbed or squeezed, but removed with an extractor that you can buy at a pharmacy. (Using your fingernails is only asking for trouble. . . they introduce bacteria that can cause inflammation.) It's tempting to pop whiteheads, blackheads, and pimples. Pimples that are infected and have yellow pus may be squeezed, but only if done properly. To do so, apply a warm compress to the area for a few minutes to open your pores, and then squeeze with a clean tissue until all the goo runs out. By doing it this way, you will allow your pimple to heal properly. And remember, washing your face more will only dry out your skin but won't improve your acne.*

AGE SPOTS (See Liver Spots)

ANXIETY

Don't panic—it's only anxiety.

When you feel worried or scared but there doesn't seem to be a clear reason, you're experiencing anxiety. Usually, our bodies go into a "fight or flight" mode when there's something to fear. But sometimes this happens when there isn't anything to be frightened about.

Being anxious is a normal response to situations of uncertainty, trouble, or feeling like you're unprepared. But if common everyday events bring on relentless and constant worry or even feelings of panic that get in your way, you may have anxiety. If this is a persistent problem, please consult your physician. However, for the person with only the occasional freak-out, here are a few remedies that might help:

A

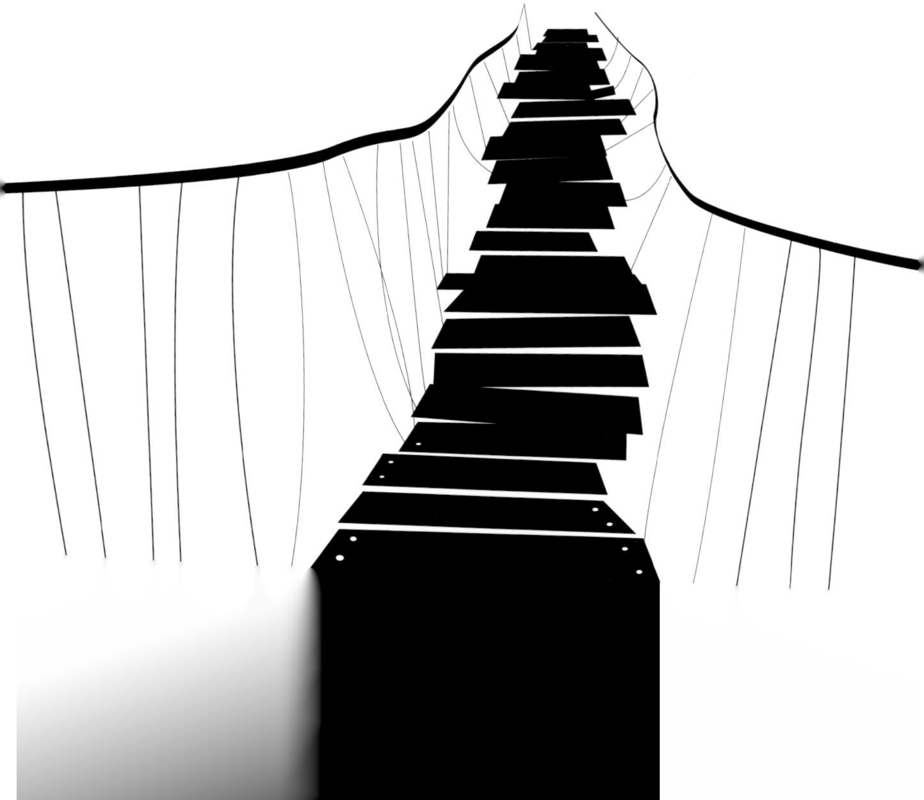

APPLE CIDER VINEGAR

- Make an anti-anxiety cocktail by putting one tablespoon of apple cider vinegar into one cup of boiling water, simmer for a few minutes, and then sip like a cup of tea. Add a teaspoon of honey to sweeten your experience.

BAKING SODA

- A warm bath with half a cup of baking soda can relax you and help to pacify your anxiety. Soak for fifteen to thirty minutes and then towel dry.

HONEY

- Eating honey is naturally calming for people who are nervous or high-strung. Eat one tablespoon of honey at bedtime–it's as yummy as it is helpful!

SALT

- In this situation, the remedy reads: "Less is definitely more." Reducing salt in your diet may potentially alleviate your bouts of anxiety.

CAUTION: *If you have anxiety every day or believe that it's related to depression, you may want to see a therapist or psychiatrist.*

ATHLETE'S FOOT

If athletes get athlete's foot, do astronauts get mistletoe?

Athlete's foot is that reddish, crackled, itchy, flaky skin between your toes that's caused by a fungus. Thriving in warm, moist places, the condition is highly contagious, and is often picked up in locker rooms, showers, public swimming pools, or other similar public areas. You can use one of the traditional over-the-counter powders or creams found at your pharmacy, or you can be a sport and try one of the remedies listed below:

APPLE CIDER VINEGAR

- To relieve your itching and peeling feet, soak them in a 50/50 mixture of apple cider vinegar and water for ten minutes daily up to ten days or until symptoms disappear.

BAKING SODA

- To prevent the reoccurrence of athlete's foot, sprinkle baking soda inside your sneakers each night.

LEMON

- While in the shower, squeeze and rub half of a lemon on each foot. Since athlete's foot is an open wound, this may sting, so be prepared!

SALT

- Add two teaspoons of fungus killing salt to four cups of warm water and soak your feet for ten to fifteen minutes and then dry thoroughly.

BAD BREATH

Bad breath stinks.

Not realizing there's a problem, your bad breath might blow others away. Unfortunately, it's a problem that's not at all unusual! If you do have bad breath, understand that certain foods and sloppy oral hygiene can cause it. Consider brushing your teeth after each meal and flossing daily. And although having bad breath stinks, here are a few things that you can do to pretty your pucker:

APPLE CIDER VINEGAR

- Add a tablespoon of apple cider vinegar to an eight-ounce glass of water and drink it down before each meal. This should freshen your breath and aid with your digestion as well.

BAKING SODA

- Brush your teeth with baking soda to help reduce the acid in your mouth. This creates an unfriendly environment for those odor-causing bacteria.

LEMON

- After eating, if brushing your teeth isn't possible, rinse your mouth with lemon juice diluted with water.

OLIVE OIL

- Swish a tablespoon of olive oil in your mouth to mop up your bacteria and carry them away.

SALT

- Gargle with warm salt water made of one teaspoon of salt added to an eight-ounce glass of warm water to clean out the bacteria that might be causing your bad breath.

CAUTION: *If in addition to having bad breath you also have pain in your mouth or throat you should be evaluated by a medical or dental professional.*

BEDWETTING

Most kids who wet their beds eventually stop. So if your child wets every night, don't be discouraged and don't worry that she or he isn't normal. Rest assured, bedwetting isn't usually caused by body or emotional problems.

Bedwetting will likely go away on its own without any treatment. But if your child has a chronic problem, it's still a good idea for you to talk to

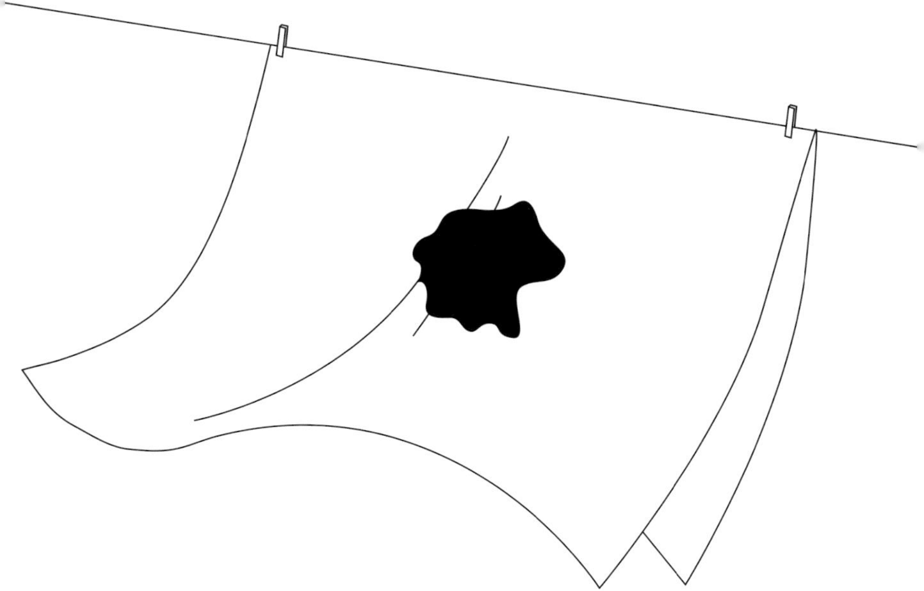

your doctor about it. In the meantime, if you live with one, leak a few of these remedies to your bedwetting child:

APPLE CIDER VINEGAR

- To limit your child's urge to urinate, mix two tablespoons of apple cider vinegar into an eight-ounce glass of water and have your child drink it with each meal. Sweeten it with some honey if the drink is too bitter.

HONEY

- If your child is over the age of one, and suffers from stress-related bedwetting, calm your child with a teaspoonful of honey at bedtime.

OLIVE OIL

- For your child's stress-related bedwetting, massage his/her belly with the smallest amount of warm olive oil before bedtime.

BLACK EYE

A black eye is a relatively common injury caused when blood collects in the space around your eye. Swollen and dark, most black eyes are minor problems, and usually heal on their own in a few days. If it's a whopper, professional medical attention should be sought.

Despite the name, "black eye," the eye itself isn't usually injured. The skin around your eye may be really discolored and bloated without any injury to the eyeball itself. It's kind of like a bruise around your eye. And like most any bruise, as a black eye heals, the swelling goes down and the discoloration gradually fades away. While you're waiting for yours to heal, hopefully you'll see clearly to try the following:

APPLE CIDER VINEGAR

- Apply a compress of equal parts of apple cider vinegar and cold water onto your bruised eye.

BLADDER INFECTION (See Urinary Tract Infection)

CAUTION: *If you are pregnant or have diabetes, you should be evaluated further by a medical professional because of the risk of miscarriage in the former and kidney infection in the latter.*

BLISTERS

Most people commonly get blisters from walking, wearing tight shoes, or from friction-burns. If you've gotten a blister, and it isn't too painful, do everything possible to keep it intact. If left unbroken, the skin over your blister will provide a natural barrier from bacteria, decreasing its risk of becoming infected. Place an adhesive bandage over your blisters after treating them with one of the following. Remember, if the right steps are taken, your blisters will be fine:

BAKING SODA

- Add enough water to a tablespoon of baking soda to make a paste and apply directly to the blister, allowing the mixture to dry. Repeat two to three times each day.

HONEY

- Applying honey directly to the blister can also aid in healing. Since the honey is sticky, cover the affected area.

LEMON

- Place a slice of lemon on your blister and leave it there as long as you can, changing often with a fresh slice. Repeat this process twice a day—morning and night.

OLIVE OIL & APPLE CIDER VINEGAR

- Apply a mixture of one tablespoon of olive oil and one tablespoon of apple cider vinegar to the affected site twice daily. Leave the mixture on for about thirty minutes and then rinse off. Any itching should be resolved immediately, and the sores should be resolved in about a week.

SALT

- Dip your moist index finger in common salt and press on the blister sore for thirty seconds. Rinse off and repeat twice daily.

BLOATING

Bloating is the swelling of your tummy area with symptoms that leave your abdomen feeling full and tight. Sometimes painful, your bloating may also be accompanied by stomach rumbling and grumbling. Instead of using your usual treatment, expand your horizons by trying one of the following:

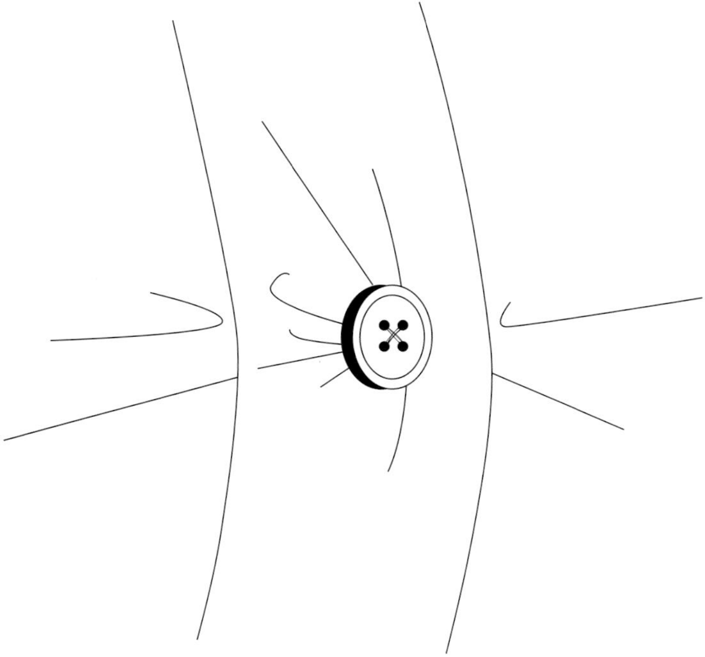

APPLE CIDER VINEGAR

- Every day, drink an eight-ounce glass of water mixed with one or two tablespoons of apple cider vinegar and you'll alleviate gas and bloating.

BAKING SODA

- A tonic of baking soda in water helps cure a gassy, bloated stomach. Mix ¼ tablespoon with a few ounces of tepid water. It's not a delicious drink, but it's worth the instant relief.

LEMON

- To relieve bloating, squeeze the juice of ½ lemon into a cup of hot water. Give it a stir, toss it back, and enjoy the results.

OLIVE OIL

- Concoct a nonalcoholic digestif! Drink plenty of noncarbonated fluids and follow with a tablespoon of olive oil to help you poo faster and easier.

SALT

- Because salt contributes to bloating, refrain from foods and drinks high in sodium and its irritating effects.

BLOCKED EAR

Lined with hair follicles and glands that produce wax, the ear canal protects itself by trapping dust and other airborne particles. Your earwax prevents most of the flotsam and jetsam of the world from entering and damaging your ear, and usually makes its way to the opening of your ear where it falls out or is removed during washing.

Some ears produce more wax than others. Unfortunately, sometimes this extra wax hardens and blocks your ear. Attempts to clean your ear with a cotton-tipped swab (oh, c'mon, you know you do it!) only push the wax deeper into your ear canal, causing further blockage.

Don't be EAR-Responsible. Never put anything smaller than your elbow in your ear! Instead, keep them wax-free and clear with the following tips:

BAKING SODA

- The easiest way to remedy your blocked ears is to make a mixture of five parts warm water and one part baking soda. Using an ear syringe, gently squirt the solution into your ear. The baking soda will loosen your hardened wax.

LEMON

- If you have blocked ears while flying, try sucking on a piece of lemon. (Of course this requires first getting the attention of your flight attendant to get the lemon.)

OLIVE OIL

- For blocked ears, olive oil can help soften the wax and enable it to come out. Apply two warmed drops in each ear twice a day.

BODY ODOR

Occasional body odor can be treated if you know the cause, and—clearly—a program of daily bathing, altering your diet, and changing your clothes regularly are logical places to begin.

Bathe yourself daily to remove bacteria—especially your armpits and groin area where germs are most prevalent. Remember to scrub your nooks and crannies with a soapy washcloth to remove any offenders. If you smell a rat when using commercial products with all those chemicals, breathe easy by applying these alternatives:

APPLE CIDER VINEGAR

- Instead of deodorant, pour apple cider vinegar on a cotton ball and apply to your underarms. The stink of the vinegar smell goes away in minutes leaving you odor-free all day.

BAKING SODA

- Use baking soda, an odor-eater, instead of deodorant. Apply the powder to your dry armpits. It'll kill bacteria and help absorb perspiration.

HONEY

- A solution of one tablespoon of honey added to lukewarm water as a rinsing solution will help keep your body odors in check.

LEMON & SALT

- Cut a lemon in half and sprinkle the fruit side with salt. Rub it on the part of your body where there is an offensive odor. You can use this on your hands if you've just chopped garlic or onions or on your underarms after a bath instead of deodorant.

BRUISES

Bumping yourself and rupturing the tiny capillaries under your skin leaves a darkened area called a bruise. For those people who bruise easily, think about taking a shine to the following remedies:

APPLE CIDER VINEGAR

- Soak a cotton ball in apple cider vinegar and apply it to the bruised area for one hour. The apple cider vinegar reduces the blueness and speeds the healing process.

HONEY

- Put a small amount of honey on your bruise and cover it with a bandage. Honey will minimize the bruise by causing your swelling to go down.

OLIVE OIL & SALT

- Place a dribble of olive oil and a sprinkle of salt onto a piece of gauze. Place the olive oil and salt covered side of the gauze over your bruise. Cover with paper towel and tape a plastic bag over area for about one to two hours. Remove and rinse off.

BURNS – MINOR

Dry heat (like fire), wet heat (such as steam or hot liquids), radiation, friction, heated objects, the sun, electricity, or even chemicals cause burns.

Before giving first aid, assess how badly burned you are. If your burn is severe, seek medical attention **immediately**.

If you have money to burn, use expensive over-the-counter treatments to care for your minor burn. If not, or if you're just a skinflint, consider the following skin treatments:

HONEY

- Honey has antibacterial properties and will promote healing. After applying honey to your burn cover the area with sterile gauze.

LEMON

- Lemon is a cooling agent and will reduce the burning sensation on your skin. Additionally, lemon juice applied on the areas of your burns can fade your scars.

OLIVE OIL

- Olive oil will bring relief to a painful burn or scald and will improve the chances of healing without a blister or a scar.

SALT

- Rinse minor burns with a saltwater solution of ¼ teaspoon of salt in eight ounces of warm water; it'll relieve the pain and minimize scarring.

CANKER SORE

Canker sores are those painful, recurring white spots that appear inside your mouth, on the inside of your cheeks, or on the edges of your tongue. It's generally believed that stress, poor dental hygiene, food allergies, and nutritional deficiencies are possible triggers for canker sores. Keep track of when you get them so you can determine ways to avoid getting them in the future.

In the meantime, give your lesions a lesson by treating your canker sores with one of the following:

APPLE CIDER VINEGAR

- Soak a cotton swab in apple cider vinegar and insert it into your mouth. Hold the swab on the site of the canker sore for one minute. Repeat several times throughout the day.

BAKING SODA

- Mix a teaspoon of baking soda with ½ cup of warm water and use as a mouthwash several times a day, especially after meals and before bedtime.

HONEY

- Apply a honey-soaked cotton swab five to six times a day to help relieve the pain of canker sores and to help them heal.

LEMON

- Lemon juice can disinfect canker sores in your mouth. Apply lemon juice diluted with water (five teaspoons of water to one teaspoon of lemon juice) to the affected areas, or gargle with the mixture several times a day.

SALT AND BAKING SODA

- At the first sign of a canker sore, gargle with a mixture of one teaspoon baking soda and a pinch of salt in a cup of warm water.

CHAFING (See Rashes)

CHAPPED LIPS

- Chapped lips are caused when your lips become dry and cracked from the evaporation of moisture, particularly in cold weather or from sun exposure. To avoid it, consider wearing a lip balm and applying it often. To maintain your beautiful smile and to "lick" your chapped lips, consider the following preparations:

BAKING SODA & HONEY

- Mix equal portions of honey and baking soda and apply this mixture onto your lips, gently rubbing it in. This paste will remove your dead skin cells and leave your lips super soft.

HONEY & OLIVE OIL

- For chapped lips, rub gently with honey and then apply a light coating of olive oil. Repeat several times a day, particularly when going outdoors.

LEMON

- Believe it or not, rubbing a slice of lemon on your lips is a useful cure if they're chapped.

OLIVE OIL

- Put a little bit of olive oil onto your chapped lips. You will have immediate results. Apply it as often as you need it.

SALT

- Treat your chapped lips with a cooling saltwater compress made by soaking a cotton ball in a mixture of ¼ teaspoon salt and eight ounces of warm water. Repeat several times a day, but always with a fresh cotton ball.

CIRCULATION

Your circulation system is the nonstop flow of your blood. It pumps oxygenated blood through your arteries to the itsy-bitsy blood vessels and every part of your body. It then flows back to your heart through your veins, only to start the cycle all over again. This uninterrupted movement of your blood is necessary to maintain the supply of oxygen from your lungs and nutrients from your gut. It's also essential for the distribution of water and heat as well as the removal of waste. The five liters of blood in a typical adult re-circulates 1,500 times each day. To boost your circulation, go with the flow and consider one of the following:

APPLE CIDER VINEGAR

- One tablespoon of apple cider vinegar mixed with eight ounces of water can help to increase your circulation.

BAKING SODA

- Take a warm bath with a cup of baking soda added. The warm water paired with the baking soda will increase your circulation.

HONEY

- Honey applied topically has anti-inflammatory properties that may also improve circulation to specific areas.

LEMON

- When applied topically, lemon juice aids in circulation and acts as an antiseptic as well.

OLIVE OIL

- Olive oil is one reason why heart and circulation-related health conditions are relatively rare in Mediterranean countries. When it comes to oils and fats, the diet in that region includes olive oil almost exclusively.

SALT

- Scrubbing with salt not only exfoliates skin, but also increases circulation.

COLD SORES

Sometimes called fever blisters, cold sores are groups of small blisters on your lips and around your mouth. The skin around those blisters is often red, swollen, and sore and may break open, leak a clear fluid, and then scab over. Fortunately, they usually heal in a few weeks. Until then, keep a stiff upper lip and try a few of the following for comfort:

APPLE CIDER VINEGAR

- Pour a few drops of apple cider vinegar on a cotton ball and apply it to your cold sores or blisters.

BAKING SODA

- For a cold sore that appears inside your mouth, make a mouthwash from one teaspoon of baking soda added to eight ounces of warm water and sip, swish and spit until you've finished the full glass. Repeat this process morning and night.

HONEY

- Apply honey when you first feel the blister coming on. It will tingle a bit, but the honey will stop the cold sore from coming out. If it's already out, applying honey will help the cold sore heal faster.

LEMON

- Lemon juice is known for its healing properties and it effectively increases the rate at which a cold sore will heal. Directly apply undiluted lemon juice over your cold sore. The lemon will also disinfect the blistered skin.

OLIVE OIL

- A dab of olive oil will keep cold sores softer, suppler, and less painful.

SALT

- Dip your clean, moist index finger in powdered salt and press it onto your sore for thirty seconds and then rinse with warm water. Repeat this remedy morning and night.

CAUTION: *If your cold sores are recurrent, the risk of transmitting herpes is high. You should see a medical provider at the first sign of a breakout to be diagnosed.*

COLDS

Viruses make computers freeze and people sneeze.

The first symptoms of a cold may include that annoying little tickle in your throat, a runny or stuffy nose, a sore throat, coughing, a headache, a mild fever, fatigue, muscle aches, loss of appetite, and/or sneezing, sneezing, sneezing. And despite whatever "old wives" tales you've heard, not wearing a jacket or sweater when it's chilly, sitting or sleeping in a draft, or going outside with wet hair *do not* cause colds.

But no matter how you caught your cold, instead of coughing it up at the drugstore register, consider trying these homemade remedies instead.

APPLE CIDER VINEGAR

- At the first sign of a cold, drink a teaspoon of apple cider vinegar in ½ cup of warm water several times.

BAKING SODA

- Getting a cold? Soak for thirty minutes in a warm, soothing bath with ½ cup of baking soda added.

HONEY

- While you have a cold, try soothing your sore throat by sipping warm water with honey.

LEMON

- Feel a cold coming on? Sip an eight-ounce glass of hot water and the juice of a lemon. Drink up every few hours.

SALT

- Make a nasal rinse by adding a pinch of salt to an eight-ounce glass of warm water. Dribble the mixture into one nostril, holding it as long as you can, and then blow it into a tissue. Follow with the other nostril. You'll notice a marked improvement in your breathing.

CONGESTION, CHEST

With a congested chest you feel tired because you can't inhale the proper amount of oxygen. Congestion produces gooey mucus as a natural response to a lung irritation, and coughing is the normal reaction for clearing the lungs and throat of that mucous. (Also see Coughs.)

If you develop a high fever or notice blood when you cough, you might have a more serious condition, like pneumonia. See your doctor immediately!

When your chest is congested, get plenty of rest until your lungs clear up. And while resting, open yourself up to the following remedies:

APPLE CIDER VINEGAR

- For chest congestion, soak a cotton ball in apple cider vinegar and wipe it across your chest, neck, ears, and throat. Repeat throughout the day.

LEMON

- To help loosen congestion and prevent dehydration, squeeze a lemon into a cup of hot water and drink every couple of hours.

SALT

- Treat coughs that accompany chest congestion with a saltwater gargle made of ¼ teaspoon of salt in eight ounces of warm water. Fill your mouth with the mixture, gargle, spit, and then rinse.

CONJUNCTIVITIS

Caused by an infection or allergy, conjunctivitis (known as "pink eye") is the most common form of eye irritation and is highly contagious. It's an inflammation of the white of the eye and inner eyelid. When your eye becomes irritated or infected, the tiny blood vessels dilate and turn red.

For comfort from conjunctivitis, envision one of the following remedies:

BAKING SODA

- For conjunctivitis, mix one teaspoon of baking soda in cup of water. This makes a really soothing eyewash.

LEMON

- Put a single drop of lemon juice into two tablespoons of boiled water that's cooled, and bathe your eyes using sterile cotton balls. Gently wipe across your lightly closed eyelids from the nose outwards, then DISCARD THE COTTON! Always use a new piece of cotton for each swipe, and be sure to wipe both eyes, even if only one is affected.

SALT

- Stir a teaspoon of salt into one cup of warm water until dissolved. Fill an eyedropper, and put two to three drops directly into your eye.

CAUTION: *(a) Conjunctivitis is very contagious, and if you have eye pain or blurred vision, you should get evaluated by a medical professional. (b) You may have an eye condition called iritis or uveitis. If you have eye pain, extreme sensitivity to light, or blurred vision, you should see a medical professional.*

CONSTIPATION

Constipation is a condition where your bowel movements aren't as frequent as you'd like them to be. Sometimes uncomfortable, your stools may be small and hard. Occurrence of bowel movements varies from person to person, "butt" regularity is the goal. For optimum health, you should have one to three good bowel movements every day. Enjoy the following—and toast by saying "Bottoms up!":

APPLE CIDER VINEGAR

- For regularity, drink two teaspoons of apple cider vinegar twice a day with an eight-ounce glass of water.

BAKING SODA

- Add ½ cup of baking soda to a warm bath. The baking soda and the warmth of the water may help you relax, and relaxing may help you make "number two."

HONEY & LEMON

- Drink an eight-ounce glass of warm water mixed with the juice of half a lemon and three tablespoons of honey every morning on an empty stomach to treat your constipation.

OLIVE OIL

- To help relieve your constipation, take one tablespoonful of olive oil in the morning and one tablespoonful an hour after dinner.

c

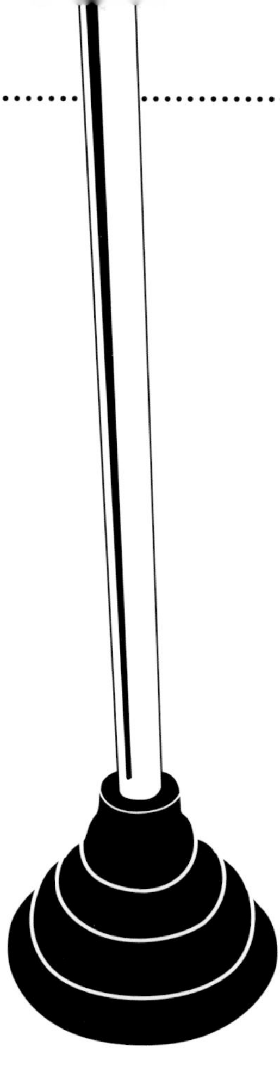

SALT AND LEMON

- Add a pinch of salt to a mixture of eight ounces of water and the juice of ½ lemon. Drink up to treat your constipation.

CONTACT DERMATITIS (See Dermatitis)

CORNS

Do only the calloused get corns?

Ill-fitting shoes produce corns. They rub your feet and toes, causing a build-up of skin and pressure on the nerves. The first thing to do is to get proper fitting shoes. For relief, put the shoe on the other foot and try these different remedies:

APPLE CIDER VINEGAR

- Soak your feet in a shallow pan of warm water combined with a half cup of apple cider vinegar. Rub down your corns with a clean pumice stone before drying. Do this again and again, day after day, until your corns are gone.

BAKING SODA & SALT

- Soak your tootsies for about twenty minutes in hot water with ½ cup of baking soda and ½ cup of salt added. Gently scrub your corns with a pumice stone. Do this every day until your corns have vanished.

LEMON

- Soak your feet in warm water for fifteen minutes, then follow up by applying a small piece of the inside of a lemon peel to your corn. Bandage it in place and leave it on overnight. Repeat daily until your corns have disappeared.

OLIVE OIL

- To soften your corns, gently rub a dab of olive oil onto them regularly three to four times a day.

COUGHS

If a pony coughs when it gets a frog in its throat, do frogs get a little hoarse?

Your body's response to inflammation or irritation in the throat, larynx, bronchial tubes, or lungs is to cough. There are two basic kinds of coughs, congested and dry, each having different underlying causes. So if yours are chesty or hacking, be "phlegm-buoyant" and try a few of the following:

APPLE CIDER VINEGAR

- To thin your mucus, throughout the day drink several eight-ounce glasses of water to which one tablespoon of apple cider vinegar has been added.

HONEY & LEMON

- Honey is one of the traditional natural remedies to alleviate a cough from bronchitis. Take ½ cup honey and the juice of a fresh lemon, stir and swallow teaspoonfuls as needed. Not only does honey soothe your tickle, it has antibacterial properties, too.

SALT

- A good, old-fashioned, saltwater gargle cuts the mucus that irritates your throat. Just a teaspoon of salt added to an eight-ounce glass of warm water is effective. Gargling with salt water can be done frequently, but spitting out the salty water after gargling is essential.

CAUTION: *If you have any of the following conditions along with your cough, see your doctor without delay because you may have an infection, or the cough may indicate the presence of a more serious health condition: (a) Your cough doesn't get better after a few days; (b) You cough up blood or bloody mucus; (c) Your mucus is yellow, brown, or green and does not improve in a few days (This indicates a possible infection.); (d) If you cough for more than three days for no apparent reason.*

CUTS & WOUNDS (See Wounds and Cuts)

CAUTION: *You may need a Tetanus shot if you have not had one in the past five years.*

CYSTS (See Acne)

DANDRUFF

Typically causing itching and flaking of your scalp, dandruff can also appear in your ears, eyebrows, and on your forehead. Itch, inflammation, waxy flakes, and fishlike scales may also indicate other skin conditions accompanying your persistent dandruff. If this is your case, consider checking with your doctor:

If you're itching to care for your dandruff yourself, there's nothing flaky about the following:

APPLE CIDER VINEGAR

- To treat dandruff, apply a mixture of 50/50 apple cider vinegar and warm water to your scalp. There is no need to rinse. Allow it to air dry.

BAKING SODA

- Add a sprinkle of baking soda to your favorite shampoo. Mix well and work into your hair and scalp. Leave it on 'til it tingles, then rinse thoroughly.

HONEY

- Smear honey onto your dandruff affected area and massage gently. Leave it on your scalp for forty-five minutes and then wash. Repeat every day for two weeks or until your dandruff is gone.

OLIVE OIL

- Olive oil helps dislodge dandruff flakes and also nourishes your scalp. Dribble it on, massage it around, and then shampoo your hair as usual.

SALT

- Before shampooing, massage your scalp with salt and then rinse.

DERMATITIS

Dermatitis is a general term used to describe an inflammation of your skin. Although the disorder can have many causes and occurs in many forms, it usually involves swollen, reddened, and itchy skin.

Dermatitis is a common condition that is neither life threatening nor contagious but that may make you completely self-conscious. Don't let your dermatitis get under your skin. Self-conscious or not, consider one of the following remedies:

APPLE CIDER VINEGAR

- For comfort, apply apple cider vinegar with a cotton ball to your rash twice a day, in the morning and before bed.

BAKING SODA

- Cool compresses soaked with tap water and baking soda will temporarily relieve your symptoms.

OLIVE OIL

- Applying olive oil to your affected skin is one of the most powerful natural remedies for reducing your rash.

SALT

- For relief from dermatitis, soak in a warm saltwater bath. Dissolve a cup of salt in warm water and soak for about twenty to thirty minutes.

DIARRHEA

With diarrhea, you'll run to the bathroom plenty. It happens when there's too much water in your bowel movements and your poop is wet and runny. Lasting usually a few days, diarrhea usually goes away on its own without special treatment.

People of all ages can get a case of the runs, but persistent diarrhea may be a sign of a more serious problem and should be treated by your doctor. Until you crack the code to your diarrhea, take it easy, drink plenty of fluids, get some rest, and consider the following for a satisfying end result:

APPLE CIDER VINEGAR

- For common diarrhea, mix two tablespoons of apple cider vinegar into an eight-ounce glass of water and sip this mixture three times a day.

BAKING SODA

- Drink a glass of water containing one-quarter teaspoon of baking soda to compensate for your lost electrolytes.

HONEY

- For adults with diarrhea, thoroughly mix four tablespoons of honey with eight ounces of water and drink.

LEMON

- Drinking the juice of a freshly squeezed lemon in a large glass of water three to five times a day may kill your diarrhea-causing cooties.

CAUTION: *(a) For pregnant women diarrhea can be dangerous because it can cause a miscarriage. If you have three loose bowels in a row, see a doctor immediately. (b) Never feed honey to a baby under one year of age. (c) If your diarrhea is persistent or your stool has pus and/or blood in it, you should be evaluated by a medical professional.*

DIGESTION

Including your mouth, esophagus, stomach, small intestine, large intestine, rectum, and anus, your digestive system is made up of a series of hollow organs joined in a long, twisting tube. It's how your body breaks down food so that can it be easily absorbed into your blood stream for nourishment. To keep your system running in tip-top condition, chew on a few of the following:

APPLE CIDER VINEGAR

- To aid in digestion, mix two tablespoons of apple cider vinegar in an eight-ounce glass of water and sip slowly during meals.

HONEY

- Dissolve a tablespoon of honey in an eight-ounce glass of warm water and then chill. Make your digestion top-notch by drinking two glasses of this sweet drink a day.

LEMON

- The acid in lemon juice may aid digestion. Squeeze it into beverages or onto food.

OLIVE OIL

- When cooking with olive oil, it mixes with other foods and may assist with your digestion.

DRY MOUTH

Perhaps not as dry as vast rolling dunes or cracked flatlands, your mouth can sometimes feel like the sand-swept Sahara. While your lack of saliva might be a common problem and a nuisance, a dry mouth can affect both your enjoyment of food and the health of your teeth. So it's important not to ignore your dry mouth.

Don't live with "cotton" mouth another cotton-picking minute. Instead, pick a remedy from the following:

BAKING SODA

- Rinse your mouth with ½ teaspoon of baking soda dissolved in an eight-ounce glass of water before meals as well as during the day to help clean and refresh your mouth.

HONEY

- A teaspoon of honey relieves most dry mouths… and it's yummy! Let it melt in your mouth and repeat as needed.

LEMON

- Sucking on the rind of a lemon often alleviates dry mouth. (Some people just think about a lemon and their mouth waters!)

SALT

- Try a warm saltwater gargle made of ¼ teaspoon of salt in an eight-ounce glass of warm water to moisten your mouth.

E

EARACHE

Earaches aren't always just in your head.

An earache is severe ear pain that begins suddenly and is accompanied by a feeling of "pressure." When developed in the absence of an infection, this pressure in your middle ear is abnormal. Earaches due to infection, however, are also frequently accompanied by a fever and may also be paired with temporary hearing loss. Please speak with your doctor if you think you may have an infection.

Try these earache remedies, and your ears will be clear as a bell:

APPLE CIDER VINEGAR

- Make a mixture of ½ teaspoon of apple cider vinegar and ½ teaspoon of water and drip a few drops of this mixture into your affected ear canal.

Then gently place a cotton ball over your ear opening so the apple cider vinegar tonic doesn't drip out. Once soothed, allow to drain.

OLIVE OIL

- Put a few drops of warmed olive oil into your aching ear and then cover it with a cotton ball. Within a few minutes it should start to feel better.

SALT

- If your earache is caused by a build-up of earwax, saltwater heated to body temperature and dribbled into your ear can relieve the pain by loosening the wax.

CAUTION: *In cases of acute ear infection, you should see your medical provider because the eardrum may also rupture due to the increased pressure behind it. If this happens, there may be pus, mucus, and some blood draining from the affected ear. When in doubt, consult with your medical provider. If you know, or even suspect, you have a perforated eardrum (a hole in it), do not put any liquid in it.*

ECZEMA

When your skin itches and becomes red and inflamed, you more than likely have eczema. Beginning in early childhood, the symptoms can unfortunately last a lifetime. Although the exact cause is unknown, it's believed to be an allergic response from your body's immune system.

Don't be caught red-handed with eczema, ease your inflamed and itchy skin with the following:

APPLE CIDER VINEGAR

- To relieve the itchiness and dryness of eczema, apply a 50/50 mixture of apple cider vinegar and water on affected areas.

BAKING SODA

- Those suffering from eczema can often find comfort in a baking soda bath. Fill your tub, add half of a cup of baking soda, and soak away.

HONEY

- Apply honey liberally over your affected areas. Let it stay for five to ten minutes and then bathe to clean up. Do this twice a day, in the morning and just before going to bed at night.

OLIVE OIL

- Olive oil works to restore the moisture in your skin and also helps the eczema to fade.

SALT

- Mix salt with a little warm water to form a thin paste. Rub this mixture onto your skin to relieve your itch. Rinse with warm water and pat dry.

EYES, DRY

Lack of humidity in your home or workplace may be the source of your dry and moisture-deprived eyes. If that's the case, soak a clean washcloth in hot water and place it over your eyes for ten minutes two times a day. This stimulates your glands to produce more oil and in turn keeps your tears from evaporating too quickly. If that doesn't work, weep for joy over the remedies below:

APPLE CIDER VINEGAR

- Drink a mixture of one tablespoon of apple cider vinegar in an eight-ounce glass of water daily and you'll notice that your eyes are less dry.

BAKING SODA

- Dissolve ¼ teaspoon of baking soda into ½ cup of warm water. Use this comforting mixture as an eyewash.

HONEY

- Simmer a cup of water and a teaspoon of honey for five minutes. Then cool. Soak a cotton ball in the liquid and apply to your closed eyes.

LEMON

- A glass of lemon water first thing in the morning can often help with dry eyes. Squeeze ½ a lemon into an eight-ounce glass of water and drink up.

SALT

- Boil one cup of water with one teaspoon of salt to make a homemade eyewash. Once cooled, apply it to your dry eyes with a clean cotton ball.

F

FATIGUE

Sometimes defined as feeling a lack of motivation to do anything, fatigue isn't the same thing as sleepiness, although when you feel fatigued, you'll often want to snooze. Some days you'll have so little energy that you'll be drowsy by lunchtime and need a nap by mid-afternoon. (Sound familiar? Nodding your head in agreement?)

Stresses of modern life, medical treatments, overworking, and poor eating habits can wear you down and cause fatigue. A few simple lifestyle changes are likely to put some pep in your step. If you're dead on your feet, get fired up by trying a few of the following:

APPLE CIDER VINEGAR

- A daily tonic of two or three teaspoons of apple cider vinegar added to eight ounces of water can help you beat your fatigue.

HONEY

- Dissolve one teaspoon of honey into an eight-ounce glass of warm water and drink to help you fend off your fatigue.

LEMON

- To battle your fatigue, simply poke a hole into a lemon and suck the juice right out. Ooh, it's sour, but boy does it work!

SALT

- If you drink ½ teaspoon of salt in an eight-ounce glass of water first thing in the morning, your fatigue symptoms may disappear.

CAUTION: *Fatigue may be a symptom of an underlying medical problem that requires medical treatment. If your fatigue is not improving, you should contact your health care provider.*

FEVER

Although your body's internal "thermostat" is set at 98.6° Fahrenheit, even when you're in good health, your temperature varies throughout the day—lower in the morning and higher in the late afternoon and at night. When something's wrong, like when you have a cold or flu, your normal temperature is simply reset a few degrees higher.

Strangely, at the onset of a fever, you may feel chilly and begin to shiver to produce heat. When your body's thermostat revs up to reach the correct temperature, you'll then begin to feel hot—or have a fever. Once your fever begins to subside, you'll probably sweat, which is your body's way of reducing your extra heat.

The next time you have a fever, go ahead and work up a sweat by trying a few of the following recipes:

APPLE CIDER VINEGAR

- Put one cup of apple cider vinegar into a warm bath and soak in it for ten to twenty minutes to find relief from a mild fever.

BAKING SODA

- To relieve a low-grade fever, bathe in a tub of lukewarm water with ½ cup of baking soda.

HONEY & LEMON

- Add the juice of one lemon and a teaspoon of honey to a cup of hot water and drink it while the brew is still hot. Repeat every two hours or until your fever subsides.

CAUTION: *For high fevers of 101 or above, do NOT soak in a hot tub—and call your physician.*

FEVER BLISTERS (See Cold Sores)

F

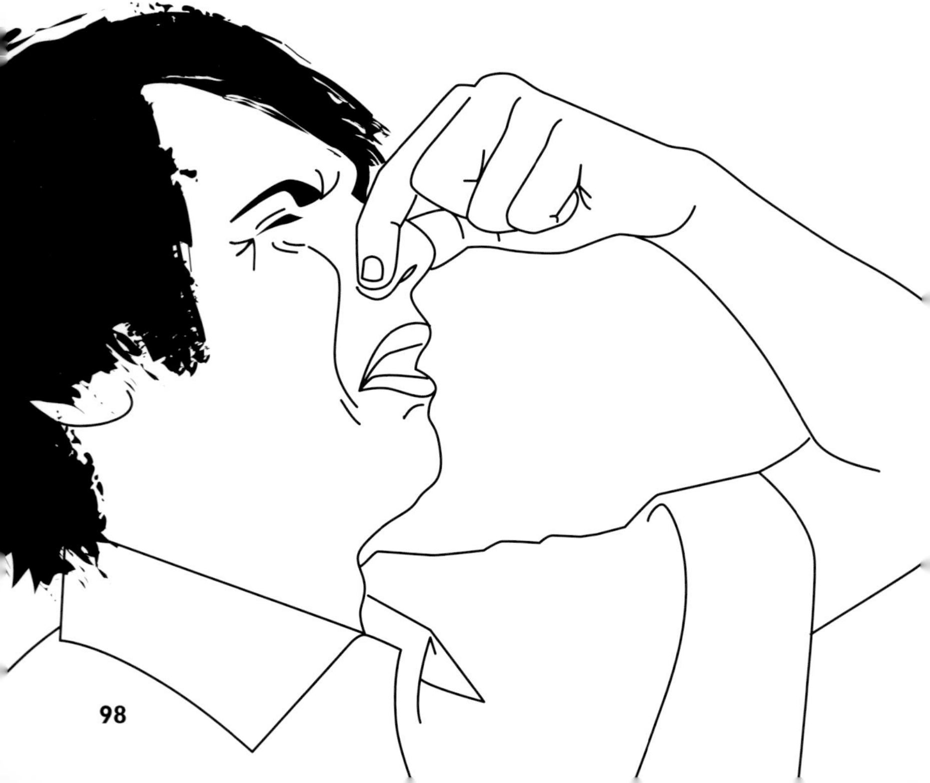

FLATULENCE

Humm-errhoids

Everyone has gas at some point in the day, and when you toot your horn, cut the cheese, or fart—you'll probably deny it. (C'mon, you know you do!) Flatulence is caused by excess gas in your stomach or intestines that builds up and needs to get out. Sometimes it makes you feel uncomfortable and bloated, and increases your tendency to belch or be flatulent.

The normal, healthy average person passes about ½ a liter of gas per day. Whether loud as a trumpet or silent but deadly, that's about fourteen farts daily. However, even though it's a natural body function, passing gas in the wrong place at the wrong time can be pretty embarrassing.

So before anyone catches wind, consider a few of the following:

APPLE CIDER VINEGAR

- Drink two teaspoons of apple cider vinegar added to an eight-ounce glass of warm water at the start of each day to reduce your need to toot.

BAKING SODA & LEMON

- Stir one teaspoon of lemon juice and ½ teaspoon baking soda into an eight-ounce glass of cool water. Drink it down quickly, right after meals. It'll force you to burp and reduce the gas build-up in your stomach.

LEMON

- Add a squeeze of lemon juice to an eight-ounce glass of water. Drinking it after meals may curtail your "barking spiders."

OLIVE OIL

- To decrease flatulence, take one teaspoon of olive oil in the morning on an empty stomach.

FLEABITES

You'll most likely get a fleabite on areas of your body where you wear tight clothing, especially your lower legs where you wear socks, and around the waistband of your pants.

With the telltale circle of red and irritated skin surrounding the small bite, fleabites itch because of your body's allergic reaction to them (though sensitivity to the bites varies from person to person).

Since dogs and cats are the main carriers of fleas, to help control them, your pets and their bedding should always be kept clean.

So if you encounter fleas, dip into one of the following remedies:

APPLE CIDER VINEGAR

- Mix one part apple cider vinegar to two parts water. Pour the mixture into a spray bottle, and spritz until your fleabites are drenched.

BAKING SODA

- Make a paste of equal portions of baking soda and water and apply it to your fleabites for relief.

LEMON

- A dribble of lemon juice on each fleabite will stop the irritation.

FOOT ODOR

Your feet sweat when you wear shoes or sneakers that don't "breathe." And after walking or exercising, when you kick your shoes off—*peeeuwww!* They stink!

Thriving in dark, damp places like the insides of sweaty shoes, bacteria are often the culprits. They usually live on your feet but also rapidly reproduce—particularly if you don't wear perspiration absorbing socks. The bacteria thrive on oils from your skin and your dead skin cells, and as their colonies grow, they get rid of their waste in the form of rotten-smelling organic acids. Besides regular bathing and laundering your sneakers, consider healing your stinky heels and toes with a few of the following:

APPLE CIDER VINEGAR

- To control foot odor, soak your feet several times a week in 1/3 cup of vinegar added to a small pan of warm water.

BAKING SODA

- Sprinkle baking soda inside your shoes, directly onto your feet, and in between your toes to absorb moisture and odors throughout the day.

HONEY

- Rub honey on stinky feet at bedtime, cover with white cotton socks, and let dry overnight. In the morning, wash with water and dry thoroughly.

LEMON

- To deodorize those "barking dogs," rub ½ a lemon onto your stinky feet.

SALT

- For super stinky feet, add ½ cup salt to four cups of warm water and soak your feet in the solution. Don't rinse; just allow them to air dry.

G

GAS (See Flatulence)

GINGIVITIS

Even if you don't have teeth, you at least have gums. And as you get older, you need to protect yours against gingivitis—the word for gum disease. With regular cleanings, brushing after meals, and flossing daily, you'll keep yours healthy and feeling fine. Don't risk a brush with gingivitis. Add a few of the following to your daily oral-cleaning routine:

APPLE CIDER VINEGAR

- Mix one tablespoon of apple cider vinegar to ½ cup of warm water and use as a mouth rinse. Sip, swish and then spit out the mixture. Repeat until you have used up the entire cup.

BAKING SODA

- Dip your finger into a solution of baking soda and water. Rub where your gums are tender or bleeding and then brush as usual.

HONEY

- Gargling with honey water may reduce the inflammation of your gums caused by gingivitis. Always rinse and then brush afterwards.

LEMON

- Add the juice of one freshly squeezed lemon to an eight-ounce glass of warm water. Use as a mouthwash, swishing it around for one minute, then spitting it out. Brush as usual.

SALT

- Try rinsing your mouth with a mixture of ½ teaspoon of salt added to an eight-ounce glass of warm water. Stir, swoosh it around in your mouth for about thirty seconds, and then spit.

GUMS, SORE

(See Gingivitis)

HANDS, COLD

(See Circulation)

HANDS, SWEATY

Because the palms of your hands have mountains of sweat glands, undue hand sweating is the most common form of out of control perspiration. And because of it, some folks have hands that sweat like crazy. Though sweaty palms can be embarrassing, they are not uncommon, and are often hereditary. Still, this condition can affect you on a functional, emotional, or social level.

Sweaty hands aren't caused by a disease; they're often triggered by emotions and stress. Current medical treatments have side effects worse than

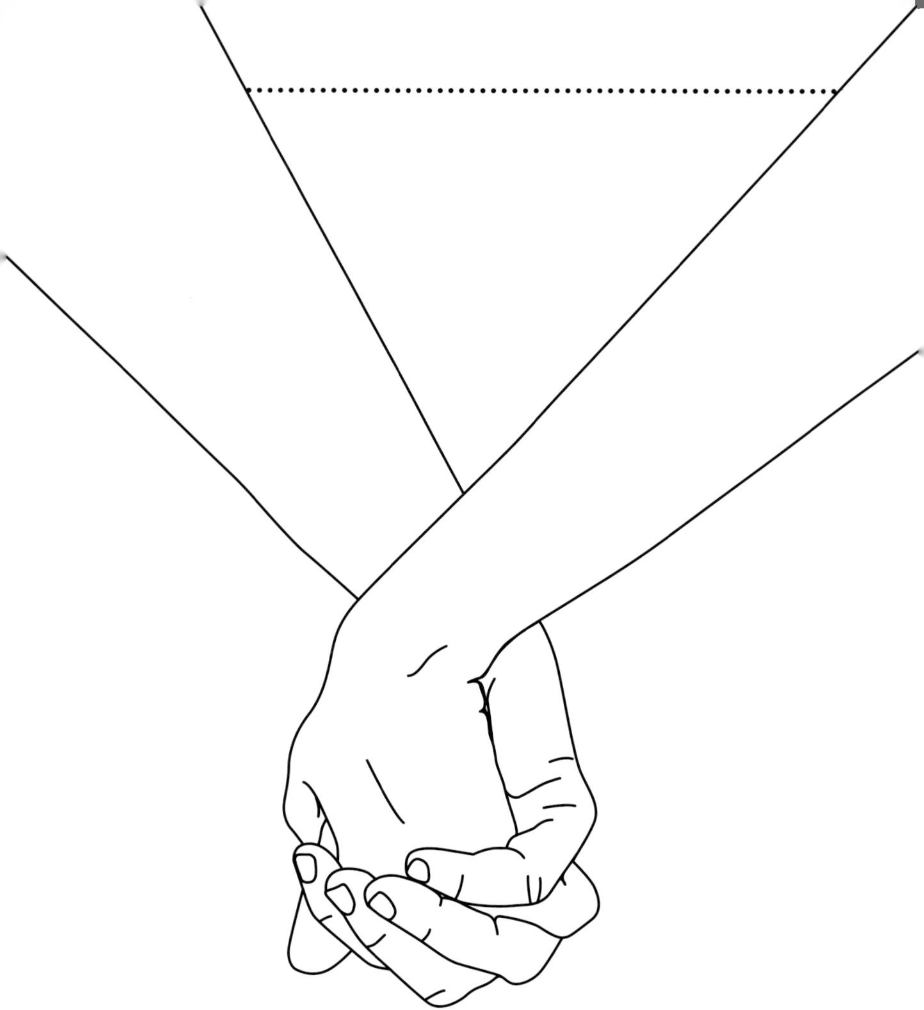

the condition itself. So keep your finger on the pulse of your sweaty hands by considering some natural and nontoxic treatments:

APPLE CIDER VINEGAR

- Wash your sweaty hands with apple cider vinegar and then rinse thoroughly. Allow to air dry.

BAKING SODA

- Try massaging baking soda into your sweaty hands and palms for five minutes and then wash thoroughly.

LEMON

- Since lemon juice has a tendency to dry the skin, soak your sweaty hands in the juice of a lemon diluted in eight-ounces of warm water. Rinse with plain warm water, then dry with a soft, fluffy towel.

SALT

- A quick treatment for sweaty hands is to soak them in lukewarm saltwater. Mix four teaspoons of salt to each gallon of warm water and soak your hands for fifteen minutes.

HANGNAILS

Hangnails aren't always a place to stash coats.

Although misleading, hangnails aren't actually part of your fingernail but are instead dead, dried-out skin. They're the sharp and barb-like pieces of flesh still attached to the base or side of your nails and are typically caused when your cuticles become dry as a bone. If you have hang-ups over your hangnails take heed of these helpful hints:

APPLE CIDER VINEGAR

- To soften your cuticles, twice a day submerge your toes/fingers in a 50/50 mixture of apple cider vinegar and water.

HONEY

- A dab of honey will soften hangnails and allow them to heal quickly. Apply and cover with a bandage.

OLIVE OIL

- Rub olive oil into your cuticles to soften them and help prevent hangnails.

SALT

- Fill up a basin or tub with warm water, add a tablespoon of salt, and soak your hands for fifteen to twenty minutes.

HANGOVERS

Hangovers often make the moon-shine brighter.

You know you have a hangover when, after a night out on the town (hell-bent on having a good time), you wake up with a pounding headache, queasiness, diarrhea, exhaustion, and aching joints and muscles. As we all know, hangovers are never as fun as the night before. So, when you can clearly

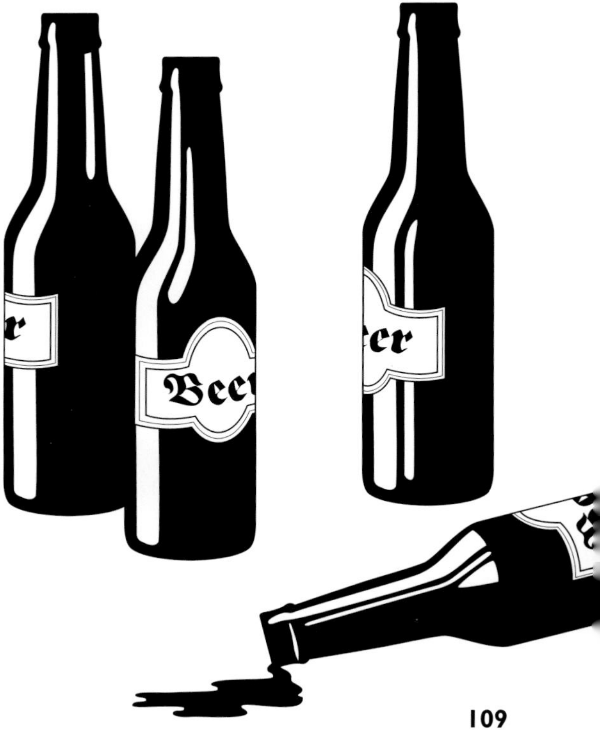
Beer

see your feet again, get a head start on healing your hangover with these tried-and-true remedies:

APPLE CIDER VINEGAR

- Apple cider vinegar is helpful with hangovers. Just pour one teaspoon of apple cider vinegar into an eight-ounce glass of warm water and drink it down immediately.

BAKING SODA

- A teaspoon of baking soda dissolved into an eight-ounce glass of water can help with the nausea associated with a hangover.

HONEY

- A tablespoon of honey before bed after you have been drinking will virtually eliminate your morning's hangover.

LEMON & HONEY

- The juice from half of a lemon and a tablespoon of honey dissolved into an eight-ounce glass of warm water is the classic remedy for a hangover.

OLIVE OIL

- A shot glass of olive oil before a night of drinking prevents a nasty hangover.

HAY FEVER

You know it by the telltale runny, red, itchy nose and eyes, but hay fever isn't caused by hay and it doesn't have anything to do with a fever. Instead, it's an allergic reaction that some folks have to seasonal allergens like pollen from plants and flowers. If you suffer from hay fever, you know that it can make you feel miserable.

Nobody else knows your nose, so only you can know if you have hay fever. When hay fever hits, these remedies should help:

APPLE CIDER VINEGAR

- Stir one tablespoon of apple cider vinegar into an eight-ounce glass of water and gulp the mixture down all at once. Do this two to three times a day for relief from your hay fever.

HONEY

- Hay-fever sufferers may find a spoonful of honey an effective remedy.

LEMON

- If you're having an attack of hay fever, squeeze half a lemon into an eight-ounce glass of warm water and drink as often as you like.

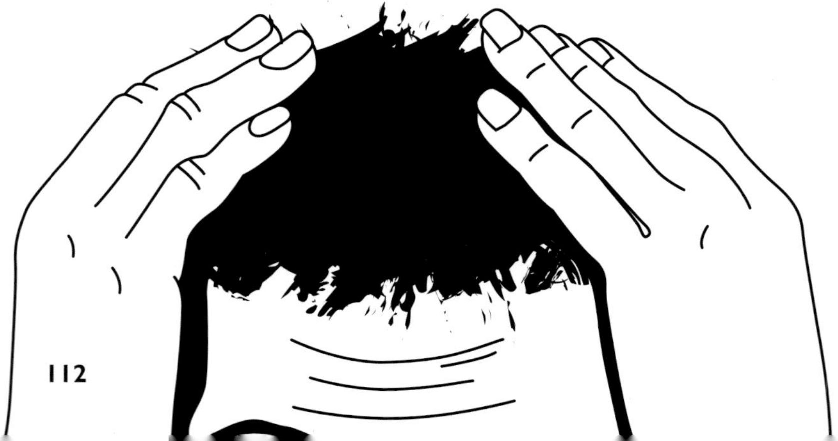

HEADACHES

Most headaches happen due to a swelling or tightening of the nerves, blood vessels, and muscles that cover your skull and neck, which then creates pressure. Those nerves send pain signals to your gray matter, and—voila—you have a headache.

Dull, continuous, and feeling as though your head is in a vise, the most common type of headache is a tension headache caused by stressed-out head or neck muscles.

Don't rack your brains looking for headache treatments; consider these:

APPLE CIDER VINEGAR

- A brown paper bag soaked in apple cider vinegar laid across your forehead often ends headaches.

BAKING SODA & LEMON

- Blend one teaspoon of baking soda with the juice of half of a lemon and warm water. Drink every fifteen minutes or until your pain begins to recede.

HONEY

- To soothe your headache, mix three heaping tablespoons of honey in boiled water and drink.

LEMON

- For a real "pounder," cut a lemon in half and then rub it across your forehead in a circular motion.

HEAD LICE (See Lice)

HEARTBURN

Spicy foods...yum! Heartburn...ouch. Eating too much food too fast or having too much caffeine are the most common causes of heartburn. Often leaving a sour or bitter taste in your mouth, the acid from your stomach gurgles up into your esophagus and makes your chest feel like it's on fire.

The next time you overdo it, don't burst into flames. Instead, try:

BAKING SODA

- Put a teaspoon of baking soda into an eight-ounce glass of water and chug it down. You'll immediately belch, and your heartburn will be relieved.

HONEY

- A teaspoon of honey quickly soothes heartburn.

LEMON & SALT

- Mix the juice of half a lemon and a pinch of salt into an eight-ounce glass of water. Drink prior to eating meals to help prevent your heartburn.

OLIVE OIL

- Take one tablespoon of olive oil on an empty stomach to relieve your nagging heartburn.

CAUTION: *See your medical provider if your heartburn is recurrent.*

HEAT EXHAUSTION

When your body overheats, you might get something called heat exhaustion. With heavy sweating and a rapid pulse, heat exhaustion comes from exposure to elevated temperatures, high humidity, and strenuous physical activity. Without speedy treatment, heat exhaustion can progress to heatstroke, a life-threatening condition.

Don't let heat exhaustion make your blood boil. As an alternative, mull over the following mixtures:

APPLE CIDER VINEGAR

- If you're suffering from heat exhaustion, apply a cool compress of apple cider vinegar and cool water to your face.

BAKING SODA & SALT

- Dissolve ½ teaspoon of salt and ½ teaspoon of baking soda in a quart of water. Lie down, elevate your feet and sip the drink to re-hydrate.

LEMON & SALT

- A squeeze of lemon and a pinch of salt added to an eight-ounce glass of cold water makes a great beverage to ward off heat stroke.

HEAT RASH

Heat rash is also known as prickly heat. Though it's most common in infants, it can actually bother anyone during hot and humid weather. It's caused when your sweat ducts become blocked and your perspiration becomes trapped under your skin. Although extremely itchy, the symptoms range from superficial blisters to deep, red lumps.

Heat rash usually goes away, but severe heat rashes may need medical care. The best way to relieve symptoms, however, is to cool your skin and prevent sweating. Give heat rash the cold shoulder by trying the following:

APPLE CIDER VINEGAR

- Add one teaspoon of apple cider vinegar to an eight-ounce glass of cool water and sponge the mixture onto the itchy areas.

BAKING SODA

- Cool off with a wet cloth dipped into a mixture of chilly water sprinkled with baking soda. Pat the affected areas of your skin.

LEMON

- Drink cool, freshly squeezed lemon juice throughout the day.

OLIVE OIL

- Applying olive oil to your affected skin is a powerful, natural remedy for reducing heat rash.

HEMORRHOIDS

Enlarged veins located in your lower "patootie," hemorrhoids are thought to be brought on by constipation and subsequent blood blockage beginning above the internal opening of your anus, which sometimes becomes swollen and protrudes. But no one really knows why some people get hemorrhoids and others don't.

Hemorrhoids often become painful from squeezing and straining when you try to move your bowels. Sometimes you sit so long, you're likely to find yourself paging through poems on the potty, jones-ing for journalism on the john, craving comics on the can, or even thumbing the thesaurus on the throne.

The next time your hemorrhoids rear their ugly heads, contemplate treating them with the following preparations:

APPLE CIDER VINEGAR & HONEY

- To stop the itching and burning of hemorrhoids, soak a cotton ball in apple cider vinegar and apply to the affected areas. Follow with a dab of honey and then cover with tissue to relieve both the swelling and the pain.

BAKING SODA

- Powder your hemorrhoids with baking soda to help stop the itching.

LEMON

- Pour the juice of ½ lemon into an eight-ounce glass and fill the rest with water. Drink this lemonade each morning on an empty stomach.

OLIVE OIL

- Drink a teaspoon of olive oil to find relief from painful hemorrhoids.

HICCUPS

A volcano is a mountain with hiccups.

Hiccups are the unexpected, unwished-for shudders of your diaphragm muscles. The hiccup sound occurs when your vocal cords snap open and shut in repeated contractions.

Safe yet annoying, hiccups can last a month of Sundays before subsiding. Instead of spazzing over your hiccups, think about a few of the following:

APPLE CIDER VINEGAR

- To rid yourself of hiccups, slowly sip an eight-ounce glass of warm water mixed with one teaspoon of apple cider vinegar.

BAKING SODA

- Add a heaping teaspoon of baking soda to $2/3$ cup of water and stir it up. Drink it all at once as fast as you can.

HONEY

- Eating a tablespoon of honey to overwhelm your mouth often puts a stop to hiccups.

LEMON & SALT

- Cut a slice of lemon and sprinkle it with salt. Savor it slowly to halt your hiccups. (I know what you're thinking; but do NOT add any tequila into the mix, or you'll end up with the hiccups all over again—and quite possibly a hangover, too!)

HIVES

Raised, red, itchy, and uncomfortable welts, hives of various sizes may appear and disappear on your skin. Commonly caused by medications, foods, or allergens, even without treatment, in most cases, hives are harmless and don't leave lasting marks.

Give your hives the heave-ho by apply one of the following:

APPLE CIDER VINEGAR

- Add a cup of apple cider vinegar to a warm bath and soak to help calm the itching cause by hives.

BAKING SODA

- Stop the itch from hives by mixing two cups of baking soda in a half-filled tub of warm water. Soak at least once a day to feel the difference.

OLIVE OIL

- Apply olive oil to your affected skin to reduce your hives.

SALT

- A salt bath (one cup of salt added to a half tub of warm water) is a superb remedy for itching cause by hives.

CAUTION: *Serious hives can be life-threatening if swelling causes your throat or tongue to block your airway, which could lead to loss of consciousness. Call 911 immediately!*

HOARSENESS (See Laryngitis)

HOT FLASHES

Hot flashes are that sudden feeling of heat across the face and upper body. In menopausal women, because your body stops producing estrogen, your inner thermostat goes on the fritz and your blood vessels go haywire, resulting in reddened skin and buckets of sweat. Eight out of ten American women experience hot flashes at menopause.

Hot flashes usually occur late in the day or after eating or drinking something hot. Hot weather and stress can also bring them on.

Fired up from flashes? Cool down with a dose of these:

APPLE CIDER VINEGAR

- To prevent flashes, massage apple cider vinegar on your chest at night.

BAKING SODA

- Draw a lukewarm bath and add one cup of baking soda. Not only will it soften your skin but it will also ease your hot flashes.

APPLE CIDER VINEGAR, HONEY, LEMON & OLIVE OIL

- Mix one cup of apple cider vinegar, one cup of olive oil, ¼ cup honey, and ¼ cup freshly squeezed lemon juice. Shake it up in a jar, pour onto your salad greens, and enjoy being hot-flash free—and well nourished!

HYPERACTIVITY

Chatty, fidgety, impulsive, unfocused, unable to enjoy quiet activities . . . or simply put—going-going-going, doing-doing-doing.

Hyperactivity (or "ants in the pants") isn't easily defined because it often depends on the viewpoint (and tolerance) of the person defining it. What seems out of control to you may not seem so to someone else. In some kids, the going-going-going interferes with schoolwork or making friends, because some are obviously more distracted than others.

"Speedy Gonzales" can use these slow but sure remedies for hyperactivity:

APPLE CIDER VINEGAR & HONEY

- To alleviate hyperactivity, take two teaspoons of apple cider vinegar mixed with one teaspoon of honey before meals.

HONEY

- Honey gives us energy without the "spike" of other sweeteners.

CAUTION: *Seek medical counsel for hyperactivity that seems to be interfering with your own or your child's ability to function at work or school, or to interact well with others. . . as it may be a sign of another, more serious, condition.*

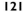

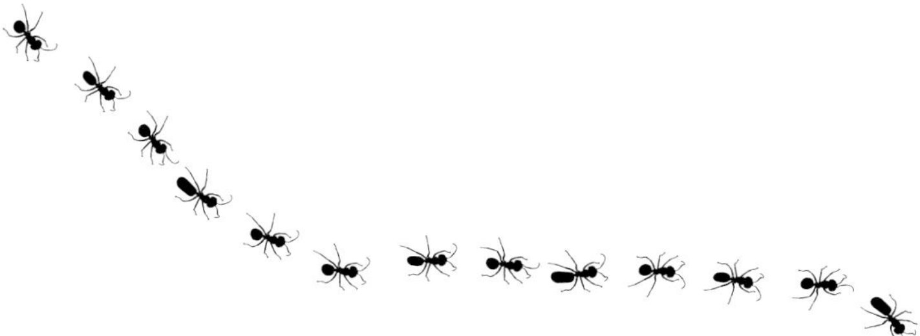

H

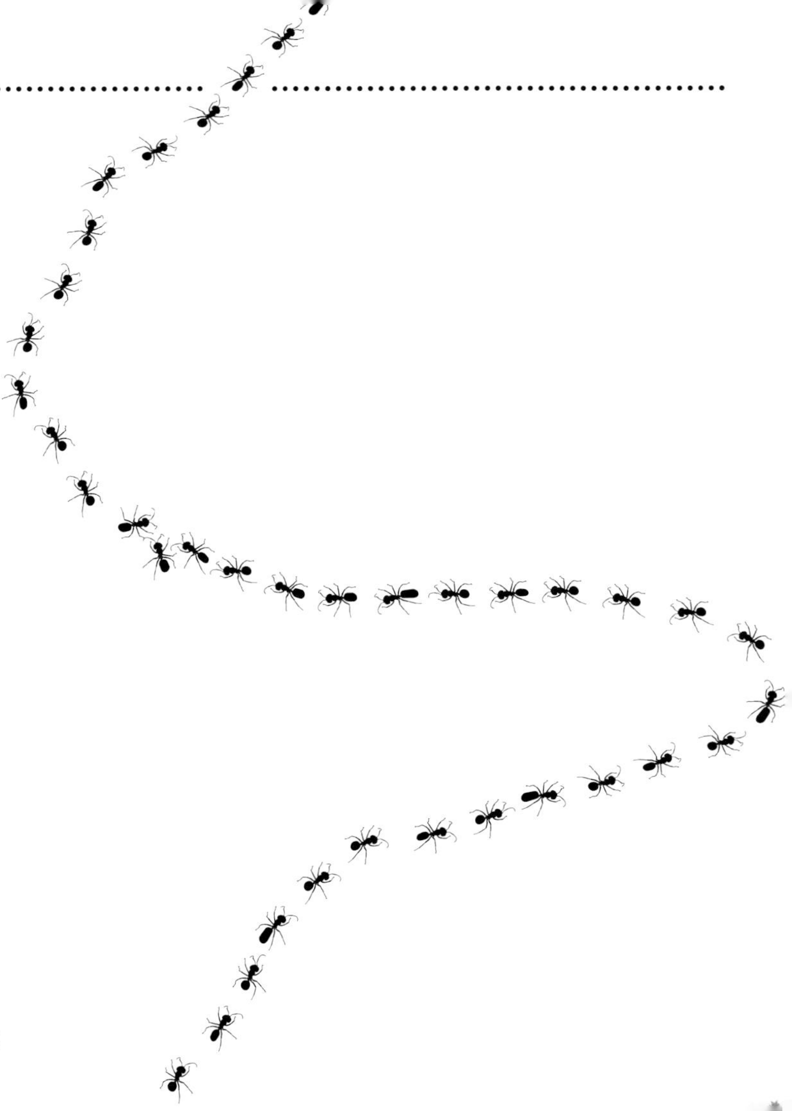

I

INDIGESTION

When you eat too much too fast, or when you pig-out on certain foods that don't necessarily agree with you, you get indigestion—just another name for an upset stomach.

Indigestion happens more frequently if you smoke, drink alcohol, are stressed out, or don't get enough sleep.

Next time you have indigestion, belly-up to a few of the following remedies:

APPLE CIDER VINEGAR

- For indigestion, drink a tablespoon of apple cider vinegar added to a ¼ cup of water.

BAKING SODA

- Drink an eight-ounce glass of warm water with a tablespoon of baking soda for instant relief.

HONEY & LEMON

- Mix one teaspoon of honey and one teaspoon of lemon juice into an eight-ounce glass of water to relieve your indigestion.

INFLAMMATION (See Swelling)

INGROWN HAIR

You have an ingrown hair when a hair curls back this-way-and-that, looping into and under your skin. While ingrown hairs commonly appear where you shave, they can naturally appear anywhere on your body, especially if you wear tight clothes.

The next time you have an ingrown hair, don't wig out. Instead, get in the loop (er... or out of it…) on simple, easy treatments:

APPLE CIDER VINEGAR

- Soak a cotton ball in apple cider vinegar; apply to ingrown hairs.

BAKING SODA

- By lightly scrubbing your skin with a teaspoon of baking soda *before* shaving, you may prevent ingrown hairs in the first place.

HONEY

- Apply honey to ingrown hairs to disinfect and soften your skin.

SALT

- Dissolve 1½ teaspoons of salt into an eight-ounce glass of warm water. Dip a fresh cotton ball into the mixture and swipe it over your ingrown hairs. Do not rinse it off; the salt mildly exfoliates and cleanses your skin, helping to draw out your hair.

INGROWN TOENAILS

Pushing into your soft tissue, an ingrown toenail hurts because it's a toenail with an edge. (Ouch!) Causing redness, swelling and pain, ingrown toenails can sometimes become infected. Improperly cutting your toenails is the main cause, but clipping your toenails flat or straight across rather than rounding the corners can help prevent the reoccurrence of ingrown toenails.

You might also get them from injuring your toes or by squeezing your feet into shoes that don't properly fit. (Note to all you fashionistas: those pretty, little, pointy-toed pumps definitely hurt sooo good—that is, until you've got a bad case of blisters, corns, or ingrown toenails!)

So, the next time you have ingrown toenails, put your foot down and slip your tootsies into these comfortable treatments:

APPLE CIDER VINEGAR

- For relief, properly trim ingrown toenails and soak in apple cider vinegar.

LEMON

- At bedtime put a lemon wedge onto your ingrown toenail and secure it in place with a bandage. By morning, the juices should have softened the inflamed skin enough to allow you to carefully trim the affected nail.

OLIVE OIL

- To minimize the pressure and discomfort, rub olive oil onto your ingrown toenail to soften your skin.

SALT

- To reduce swelling and relieve tenderness, soak your ingrown toenails for fifteen to twenty minutes three times a day in a solution of four teaspoons of salt per gallon of warm water. Place cotton under the ingrown edge after each soaking to help the nail grow properly. Allow to air dry.

INSECT STINGS & BITES

Insects such as honeybees, wasps, hornets, yellow jackets, and fire ants are some of the most common pests that sting when they're ticked off. If you're stung, the site will feel hot and itchy.

Wasps and bees can sting over and over because they're able to retrieve their stinger without injuring themselves. Honeybee stingers unfortunately rip out as they fly away, and as a result, they die.

The other common and possibly most annoying biting insect is the mosquito. You're at high risk of being bothered by their bites, but low risk of getting diseases (such as West Nile virus, malaria, and dengue fever)—and you're more likely to be bitten at dusk and dawn.

When flying insects bug you, here are home remedies to ease your itch:

APPLE CIDER VINEGAR

- Repel mosquitoes by spraying or rubbing undiluted apple cider vinegar onto your exposed skin.

APPLE CIDER VINEGAR & LEMON

- Dab equal parts of apple cider vinegar and lemon juice onto your bite or sting every five minutes until your pain disappears.

BAKING SODA

- To soothe stings, make a paste of one teaspoon of baking soda and one teaspoon of water and apply it to your sting. Leave the paste on for fifteen to twenty minutes, and then wash rinse off.

HONEY

- Ironically, applying honey immediately after being stung by a bee will keep you from having any pain.

OLIVE OIL

- Apply just a drop of olive oil for relief from stings and other insect bites.

SALT

- Apply a saltwater solution made of ¼ teaspoon of salt and eight-ounces of warm water over your bite to help relieve your itch.

CAUTION: *If you experience an allergic reaction from a sting, such as difficulty breathing or swallowing, nausea, or chest pains, go to the ER immediately. If you have antihistamines, take some. This will help reduce your reaction, but you must go to the hospital! Don't drive yourself!! Call a friend, 911, or the police. This type of allergic reaction can be fatal.*

INSOMNIA

Less rest makes insomniacs restless.

Tick-tock, tick-tock, tick-tock...*yawwwwn.* When you're having trouble falling or staying asleep—tossing and turning, this way and that—you're experiencing something called insomnia. The result is waking up feeling un-refreshed, which can then impact your ability to function during the day. And zapped of your energy, you'll probably feel weak and crabby.

Let insomnia be your wake up call. Simple changes in your daily habits may be required to restore your needed rest. Starting with these remedies may help you get your zzzzs:

APPLE CIDER VINEGAR

- One teaspoon of apple cider vinegar before bed will have you sleeping better than ever.

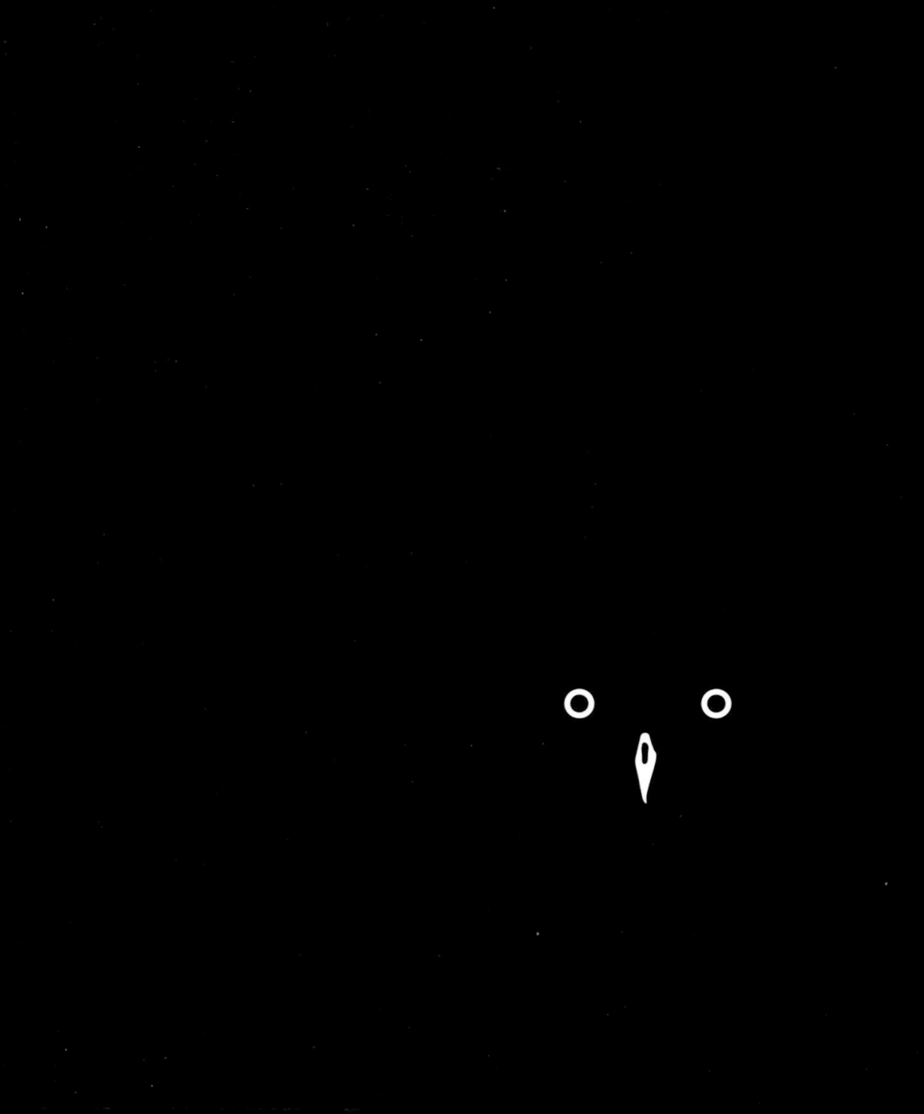

BAKING SODA

- Half a cup of baking soda dissolved into your bath before bedtime may soothe your nerves and thus help you get some sleep.

HONEY & LEMON

- Mix a teaspoon each of lemon juice and honey into an eight-ounce glass of warm water and sip before getting into bed.

OLIVE OIL

- Settle a busy mind before bed by massaging your feet a few minutes with a dribble of olive oil. Wipe the oil off when finished.

SALT

- By reducing your salt intake, you'll find yourself getting better sleep.

ITCHY SKIN (See Eczema)

JET LAG

Lagging jets rarely create jetlag.

Jet lag is when your internal clock is out of whack—usually when you fly across time zones. Wiped out, dazed, and nauseous, these temporary symptoms may throw a wrench into your vacation or business travel.

Don't leave your health up in the air. Consider these "plane" and simple remedies to help prevent or minimize it:

APPLE CIDER VINEGAR & HONEY

- Heat equal portions of apple cider vinegar and honey at home, and carry on board in a travel-size plastic jar. Add a small amount of this potion to water you drink while in flight.

(Note: be prepared to explain your elixir to airport security, should they ask.)

BAKING SODA & SALT

- To rid your body of the toxins from flying, dip into a bath containing one cup of salt and one cup of baking soda when you arrive at your destination.

JOCK ITCH

Jock itch affects the inner thighs, keester, and nudie bits, causing itchy red rashes in these warm, moist spots. Athletes get jock itch because they end up spending a lot of time in sweat-soaked shorts. But anyone—athlete or not—can get it. Fortunately, however unpleasant and bothersome, jock itch usually isn't serious.

Don't be "penile-ized" for jock itch. Keep your groin clean and dry, and score points with a few of the following:

APPLE CIDER VINEGAR

- Wash the affected areas and dry them completely. Follow by applying a 50/50 solution of apple cider vinegar and water to your jock itch twice daily. Allow to thoroughly air dry.

BAKING SODA & LEMON

- To relieve the itch that often accompanies this condition, relax in a bath with ½ cup baking soda and ½ cup of lemon juice. Towel dry.

SALT

- Immerse yourself in a bath that's been sprinkled with an entire cup of salt. Soak for fifteen minutes and towel yourself dry.

LARYNGITIS

Whinny about laryngitis or be forever hoarse.

Shouting, singing, shrieking, or speaking can sometimes lead to laryngitis, and so can a viral infection. Either way, the result is an irritation that interferes with your vocal cords. The sudden swelling causes the sounds from your mouth to distort and, as a result, your voice is reduced to a whisper. (You may not be able to speak clearly, but you'll certainly have hoarse-power!)

If your vocal cords are harmed and a persistent sore throat nags you, try these to treat yours:

APPLE CIDER VINEGAR

- Mix one teaspoon of apple cider vinegar into four ounces of water and sip to take care of your laryngitis.

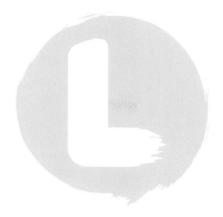

HONEY & LEMON

- Mix equal portions of honey and lemon to soothe your throat.

SALT

- Make a saltwater gargle by adding ¼ teaspoon of salt to an eight-ounce glass of warm water and gargle away. For relief from your laryngitis, do this several times a day.

LEG CRAMPS

Leg cramps, caused by an uncontrolled tightening of your muscles, can result in the out-of-control pain and momentary helplessness that often occurs as you're drifting off to sleep or just waking up.

If you're knee-deep in leg cramps, try the following:

APPLE CIDER VINEGAR

- To minimize your leg cramps, mix two teaspoons of apple cider vinegar into an eight-ounce glass of water and drink before each meal.

BAKING SODA

- Mix ¼ teaspoon of baking soda with an eight-ounce glass of water and drink it before strenuous exercise or activity.

LEMON & SALT

- Combine the juice of half a lemon with a pinch of salt into an eight-ounce glass of water for quick relief from leg cramps.

OLIVE OIL

- To relieve the cramp, rub your legs vigorously with a tiny bit of olive oil.

LICE, HEAD

Brown or gray and no bigger than a sesame seed, lice survive off other living things. Eating tiny amounts of your blood, head lice need warm skin to survive. While setting up shop in your hair, they'll lay eggs. And although lice don't hurt, your skin may become irritated and itchy.

The next time you notice them, get to the root of your head lice by brushing up on the following treatments:

APPLE CIDER VINEGAR

- At bedtime wet your head with apple cider vinegar and wrap it in a vinegar-soaked towel. Cover with yet another dry towel leaving it in place overnight. In the morning, wash your hair. The lice eggs should fall out during shampooing. Rinse and repeat the routine daily until the lice are gone. Because apple cider vinegar may stain light fabrics, it's best to use old or darker colored towels for this remedy.

BAKING SODA & OLIVE OIL

- Saturate your hair with olive oil, cover it with a shower cap, and leave it in place overnight. In the morning, shampoo with baking soda and repeat daily until the lice are all gone.

SALT

- Rinse your head with a saltwater mixture of ¼ teaspoon of salt and eight-ounces of warm water. Salt water is a natural antiseptic and will help kill the live lice.

LIVER SPOTS

Yellowish or brown, liver spots are the result of old age, a nutritional deficiency, or from too much fun in the sun. Since they take forever to develop, they take almost as much time to remove. Be persistent…try a remedy for a few months, and if your flat spots that look like large freckles aren't gone, try another one.

If too much time in the sun has left you overshadowed with liver spots, reflect on a few of the following:

BAKING SODA

- To lighten age spots, blend baking soda with water into a paste and apply it to those areas. Gently scrub for one minute and then allow the paste to air dry before rinsing it off.

LEMON & OLIVE OIL

- Dab fresh lemon juice onto your spots twice daily. Finish by moisturizing your hands with a drop of olive oil and warm water.

MENSTRUAL CRAMPS

Menstrual cramps are the annoying, monotonous, monthly aches and pains that occur in the lower abdomen that most women know all too well. For some, the tenderness is merely aggravating and for others, it can be painful enough to get in the way of your day-to-day activities

Apply a few of the following suggestions and, in a relatively short period of time, you'll be able to make your "time of the month" more bearable:

APPLE CIDER VINEGAR & HONEY

- At the earliest signs of menstrual cramps, drink a mixture of two teaspoons of apple cider vinegar and one teaspoon of honey in eight ounces of warm water for quick relief.

M

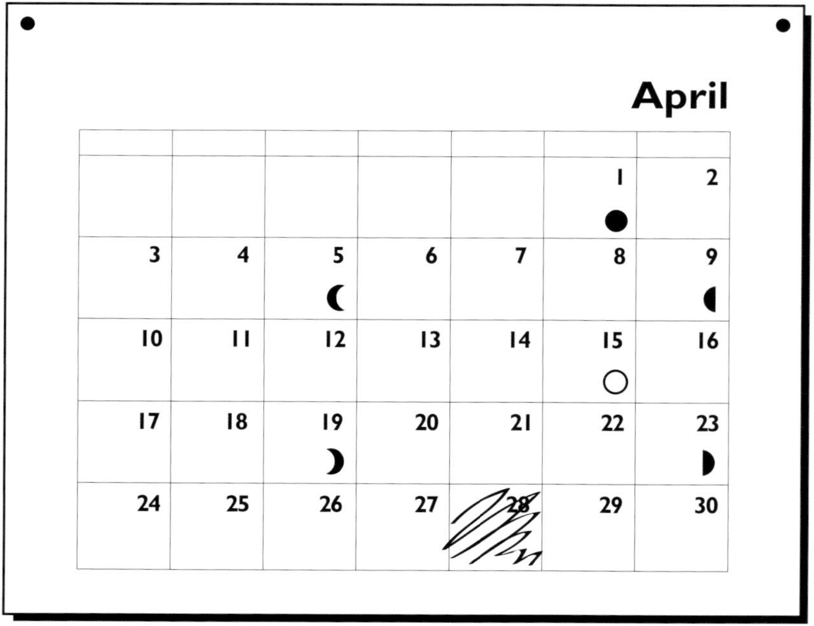
April
1 2
3 4 5 6 7 8 9
10 11 12 13 14 15 16
17 18 19 20 21 22 23
24 25 26 27 28 29 30

BAKING SODA & SALT

- Create a relaxing bath by adding one cup of salt and one cup of baking soda into a tub filled with water. Stir well 'til dissolved, then soak for twenty minutes to relieve your aching muscles and cramps.

OLIVE OIL

- Rub a drizzle of warmed olive oil onto your abdomen and massage it lightly to soothe your cramps.

MENSTRUATION

Lasting from three to five days, menstruation (also called a "period") is a woman's monthly bleeding. Menstruation is the shedding of the womb's lining. Menstrual blood moves from the uterus through the cervix, and passes out of the body through the vagina. Here are a few ideas to make the monthly visit from your "friend" more comfortable:

APPLE CIDER VINEGAR

- Taking two teaspoonfuls of apple cider vinegar three times a day with meals will hopefully minimize menstrual cramping.

LEMON

- In the case of excessive menstruation, add the juice of one lemon to a glass of cold water and drink it down to help keep your period in check.

MIGRAINES

Migraines can wipe a person out with symptoms so intense all you can think about is crawling into a darkened hole with your hands over your eyes and ears.

Affecting both women and men, these painful headaches go hand in hand with flashes of light, blind spots, tingly arms and legs, queasiness, vomiting, and an acute sensitivity to light and sound, leaving most folks out of commission for hours if not days.

If you've seen a doctor in the past and had no success in treating your migraines, it's time to make another appointment. But until then, store these curatives for relief in the back of your brain:

APPLE CIDER VINEGAR & HONEY

- For relief of your migraine, boil one cup of honey and one cup of apple cider vinegar and inhale the vapors.

HONEY

- Take two teaspoons of honey with each meal to assist in managing your migraine pain.

LEMON

- Pound lemon rinds into a fine paste and then apply it to your throbbing forehead and temples. Of course, if your migraine is already in full swing, you'll probably want and need someone else to do the pounding.

SALT

- After adding ¼ teaspoon of salt to an eight-ounce glass of water, drink to minimize the pain from your headache.

MOLES

Gorging molasses won't make moles on cute asses.

Moles are those bunches of pigmented cells that often emerge as little, murky brown spots that can grow just about anywhere on your body. Mostly harmless, inspecting moles and other pigmented areas is the first important step in detecting more serious conditions.

Instead of becoming a worrywart, here are a few suggestions on how to care for your annoying but otherwise healthy moles:

APPLE CIDER VINEGAR

- Soak your moles in warm water for fifteen to twenty minutes and then dry them off with a soft cloth. Continue by applying apple cider vinegar with a cotton ball and leave it on for ten to fifteen minutes. When finished, wash off with water and dry. This will slowly help minimize them.

HONEY

- Apply honey directly onto your moles morning and night until they have completely disappeared.

LEMON

- Gently rub whole strength lemon juice on to your moles. Repeat two or three times daily to help reduce them.

CAUTION: *Some moles may require medical attention. If you are unsure, better to be safe than sorry, so have your health care provider check them for you.*

MOTION SICKNESS

Do you feel green at sea? Want to heave while riding in the car? Feel woozy while flying? These are all symptoms of motion sickness—an ordinary interruption of the inner ear that's caused by constant motion. Simply explained, your inner ear senses an imbalance and your world then becomes topsy-turvy.

Applied with a bit of wiggle-room, these remedies should help:

APPLE CIDER VINEGAR & HONEY

- Avoid motion sickness by mixing one tablespoon of apple cider vinegar with one tablespoon honey in water and drink before hitting the road.

LEMON

- Suck on a lemon wedge to alleviate your impulse to puke.

MUSCLE ACHES (See Aching Muscles)

N

NAIL INFECTIONS

Fungus may cause infections in and around toenails and fingernails, and are an ordeal to treat. Like athlete's foot (foot? I've got two feet!), nail fungal infections occur when your tootsies or digits are exposed to the unpleasant and unsanitary conditions frequently found in places like locker rooms, pools, or even manicure and pedicure parlors. While they look—and smell—ominous (and often come with serious side effects), commercial preparations can't lay a finger on the following remedies:

APPLE CIDER VINEGAR

- Soak your affected nails for fifteen minutes a day in a basin containing two quarts of warm water and one cup of apple cider vinegar. Dry with a hair dryer set to warm.

BAKING SODA

- Create a paste by mixing baking soda with a little water and apply it all over your infected nails. Allow to air dry and repeat every morning until the fungus has completely vanished.

HONEY & APPLE CIDER VINEGAR

- Fungal infections of your fingernails or toenails can be eliminated using vinegar and honey. Dissolve one tablespoon of each into a glass of water and drink once per day.

LEMON

- Because lemon is a natural antiseptic, lemon juice can help to remove bacteria often associated with nail infections.

NASAL CONGESTION (See Stuffy Nose)

NAUSEA

Nausea ad nauseum can be nauseating.

That uneasiness in the pit of your stomach that often happens right before you puke is called nausea. Vomiting, whether intentional or involuntary, is the violent ejecting of your last meal, up from your stomach and out your mouth. There's nothing pleasant about the experience; retching is simply wretched! So the next time you feel like you need to "throw up," try some of these helpful ideas as food for thought:

APPLE CIDER VINEGAR

- To avoid or treat nausea, combine one tablespoon of apple cider vinegar in eight ounces of cold water and drink it right down.

BAKING SODA, HONEY & SALT

- Mix two tablespoons of honey, ¼ teaspoon of salt, and ¼ teaspoon of baking soda to four cups of cold water to keep hydrated while experiencing nausea—and after, too.

LEMON

- You may suck on a lemon wedge if experiencing nausea, but merely smelling a freshly cut lemon can also be super helpful.

NOSEBLEEDS

Nosebleeds can be caused by colds, allergies, dry conditions, heat, high altitudes, injuries, medications, sinus problems, and even from blowing your nose. In the event that you get a real gusher, think quickly and apply any one of these antidotes, ripe for the picking:

APPLE CIDER VINEGAR

- Soak a small cotton ball in apple cider vinegar and pack it lightly into your bleeding nostril. The vinegar will help your blood congeal.

BAKING SODA & SALT

- Spray a cold saline solution into your nose. Make it by combining one teaspoon of salt and one teaspoon of baking soda in two cups of water.

LEMON

- Put a drop or two of whole-strength lemon juice into your affected nostril to end your bleeding.

OLIVE OIL

- Swabbing your nostrils with olive oil each night may prevent nosebleeds from occurring.

CAUTION: *Call your doctor if you have blood flowing from both nostrils or if the bleeding hasn't stopped after thirty minutes. In the presence of hypertension, nosebleeds should be evaluated.*

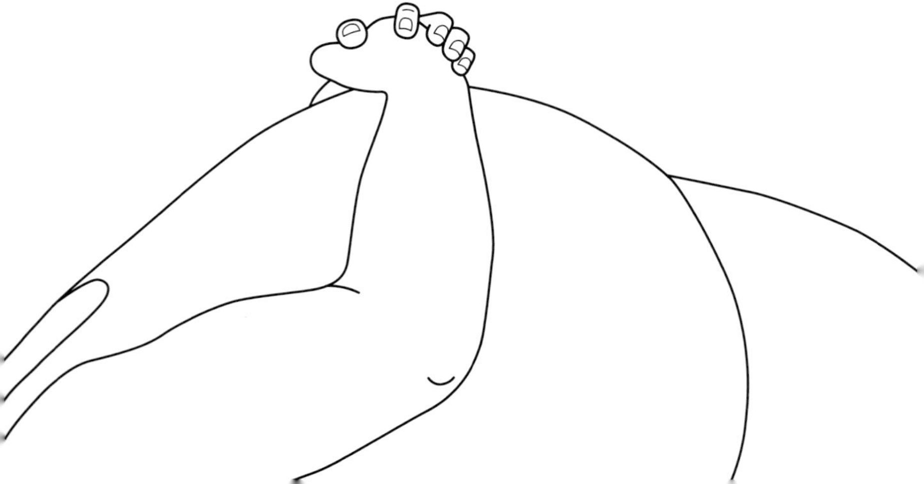

OVEREATING

Overeating takes the cake.

Overeating can mean that you either eat a lot every once in a while or …that you eat too much all the time. Either/or, overeating can cause bellyaches. The next time you overindulge, mull over these mindful remedies to find some soothing comfort:

APPLE CIDER VINEGAR & HONEY

- In the event that you overeat, take two tablespoons of apple cider vinegar in an eight-ounce glass of water. Add honey to taste. Toss it back for relief.

BAKING SODA & LEMON

- Imbibe a cup of warm water with the juice of half of a lemon and a pinch of baking soda to take the edge off that "stuffed" feeling after a big meal.

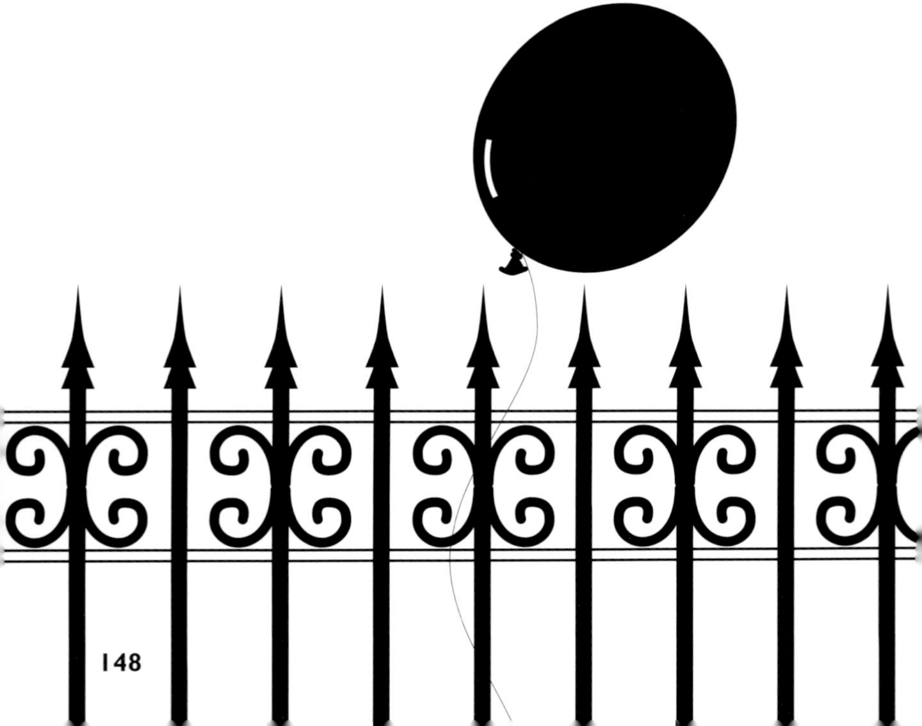

PANIC ATTACKS

Often developing for no apparent reason, a panic attack is a sudden episode of fear. Usually triggered by physical reactions, panic attacks can be terrifying because you think you're losing control of your self-control.

Although some experience only a few in their lifetime, here are a few ideas to help you calm your panic attacks and temporarily steady your world:

APPLE CIDER VINEGAR & BAKING SODA

- Dissolve two tablespoons of apple cider vinegar and ¼ teaspoon of baking soda into a half glass of water. Taken once each morning and evening, it should help calm your nerves.

LEMON

- Enjoy a cup of hot water and a slice of lemon for panic and anxiety relief.

P

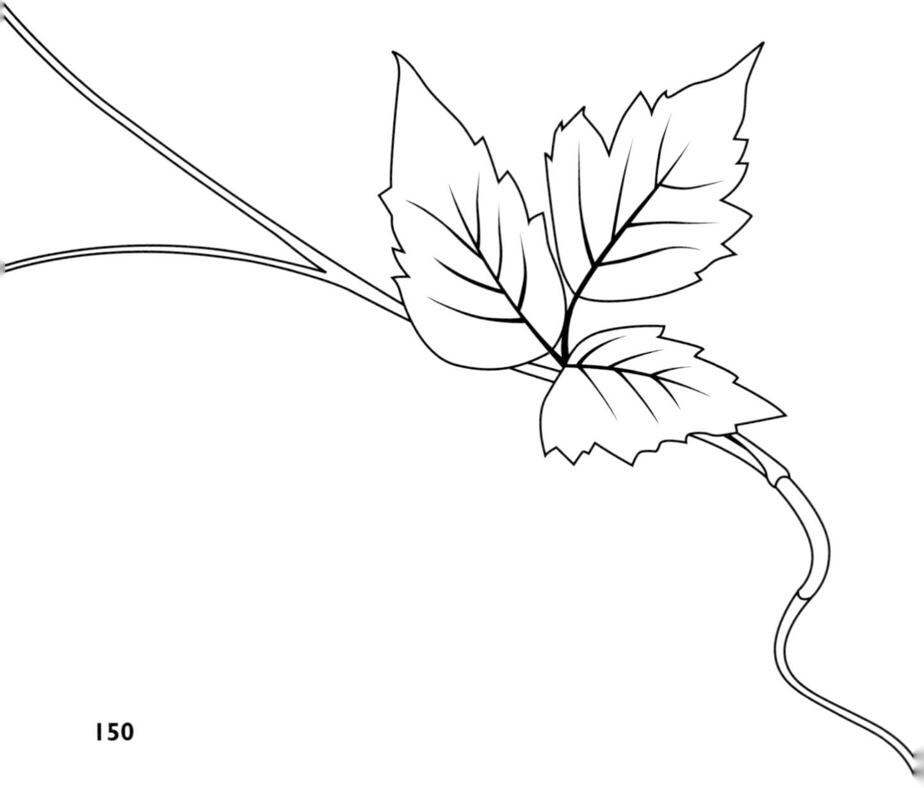

PIMPLES (See Acne)

PINK EYE (See Conjunctivitis)

PLANTAR WART (See Warts)

POISON IVY & OAK

The oil in poison ivy and poison oak is what causes the itching and blistering when you're exposed to it—and just know, the condition is gonna' get worse before it gets better. If the itching you're experiencing is mind-boggling, run very warm water over the affected area. After those poison ivy or poison oak blisters appear, wrap them with spotlessly clean bandages to avoid infection. And consider these "made from scratch" guidelines for soothing your rashes:

APPLE CIDER VINEGAR

- Use apple cider vinegar to relieve the red, itchy rash that both poison ivy and poison oak cause. Apply it liberally to the affected areas several times a day with a cotton ball or sterile gauze pad. And always was your hands thoroughly afterwards.

BAKING SODA

- Turn baking soda into a paste by adding a little water and applying it directly onto the rash. Baking soda is a good drying agent.

LEMON

- Rinse your affected areas with the juice of a lemon.

SALT

- Bathe the affected areas with a warm solution of salt water.

POST-NASAL DRIP

Sometimes caused by pollution or infections, post-nasal drip is the annoying gooey phlegm in the back of your throat that replaces your normally occurring healthy nasal secretions. Post-nasal drip is often unpleasant—and almost always irritating to those around us as we sniffle, blow, and honk in an attempt to try to get rid of it.

To dry up your dripping sinuses and get them back to normal, apply some of these treatments—they won't be any skin off your nose:

APPLE CIDER VINEGAR

- For post-nasal drip, use a solution of warm water and one tablespoon of apple cider vinegar. Place a small amount in the palm of your hand, block one nostril, and place the other nostril into the apple cider vinegar mixture and sniff hard. Let the solution run down the back of your throat and then spit it out. Repeat with the other nostril.

BAKING SODA & SALT

- Mix one teaspoon of salt and a pinch of baking soda into eight ounces of

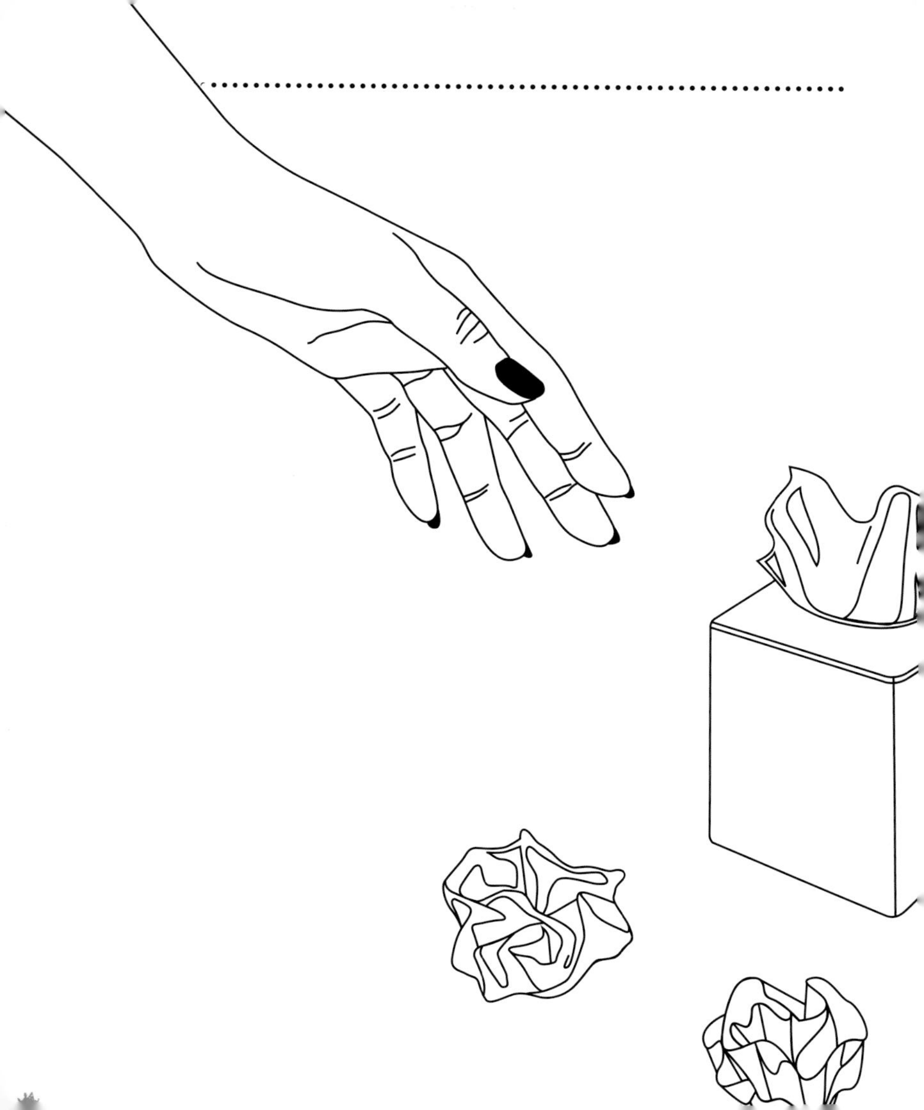

warm water. Using a nasal syringe, squirt the mixture into each nostril and then follow by blowing your nose. If you don't have a bulb syringe, you can snort the mixture out of your cupped hand.

HONEY

- While it won't actually stop the drip, a tablespoon of honey in a cup of hot water can effectively ease the pain of the sore throat that sometimes accompanies post-nasal drip.

LEMON

- To find relief from post-nasal drip, drink lots of fluids, including warm water with plenty of lemon.

PUNCTURE WOUND (See Cuts and Wounds)

R

RASHES

Resistant to the attacks of everyday life, your skin is surprisingly strong but still vulnerable, and many things can cause a skin rash—fungus, medications, parasites, viruses, or even heat.

Though not life-threatening, rashes can be unpleasant and are often a real pain in the neck. But don't be rash! Use a few of these remedies to make your outbreaks more tolerable:

APPLE CIDER VINEGAR

- Apply a 50/50 solution of apple cider vinegar and water to any rash to reduce the redness and irritation.

BAKING SODA

- To comfort a rash, add a half-cup of baking soda into a bathtub filled with warm water. Soak in the tub for thirty minutes and finish by toweling dry.

HONEY

- Dab honey on wet, weepy rashes, and cover with sterile bandages.

LEMON

- Lemon juice is effective for easing irritating skin rashes. Apply it full-strength and allow it to dry.

OLIVE OIL

- Applying olive oil to your affected skin is one of the most powerful natural remedies for reducing a rash. Wipe it on and allow it to soak right in.

SALT

- At bath time, fill your tub as normal and then pour in one cup of salt. Soak for thirty minutes, then towel dry.

RAZOR BURN

We've all done it—dragged a razor over our face or other body part only to leave behind an inflamed skin irritation caused by a blunt blade, lousy technique, or an unfortunate lack of lubrication. Razor burn can be caused by shaving too closely, shaving with a dull razor blade, not using any shaving cream, by being too aggressive, by shaving too fast or too gruffly, or by simply not paying attention at all.

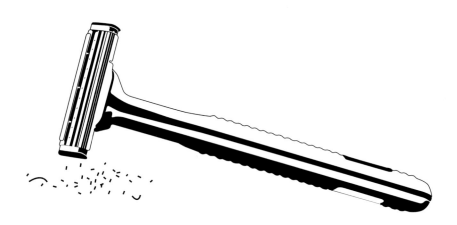

You can prevent razor burn by keeping your skin moist, using plenty of lather, shaving with the hair and not against it, and by not shaving too closely or forcefully. Perhaps the best prevention, however, is steering clear of products that annoy your skin in the first place. If you still manage to get razor burn, perhaps one of the following recommendations will make razor burn nothing more than a close shave:

APPLE CIDER VINEGAR

- Pat the affected area with whole strength apple cider vinegar and allow it to air dry.

BAKING SODA

- For instant relief, dab on a 50/50 baking soda and water solution. Allow it to air dry and then rinse it off with cool water.

HONEY

- Honey is a swell home-remedy for razor burns. Lightly cover the burn until cooled and then rinse with warm water.

OLIVE OIL

- Using olive oil instead of creams or gels while shaving may help to reduce your razor burn.

S

SINUS HEADACHE

That muffled, cavernous pain in the front of your head and face might just be a sinus headache caused by the swelled sinus passages right behind your eyeballs, cheeks, and nose. Often worse in the morning and better by afternoon, simple movements can sometimes worsen your soreness. Ponder the following to go head-to-head with your pain:

APPLE CIDER VINEGAR

- Add an eighth of a cup of apple cider vinegar into a cool-air vaporizer and inhale the infused-air directly for five minutes. Follow by lying down for twenty minutes while your sinuses clear.

BAKING SODA & SALT

- Combine ¼ tablespoon of baking soda and ¼ teaspoon of salt to a half cup of lukewarm water and mix together well. Proceed by closing your left nostril, pour a little of saltwater mixture into your right hand and snort in some of the mixture. Repeat the process with your other nostril. Drain by blowing your nose.

LEMON

- Some headaches are caused by dehydration. Drink a glass of water with a lemon twist to help your body re-hydrate.

SNEEZING

Blessings are nothing to sneeze at.

Wintry air, black pepper, dirt, filth or grime—just about anything can rub the inside of your nose the wrong way. A sneeze occurs when the interior of your snout gets a prickle or an itch, speeding a memo to your brain. Once received, your muscles work in tandem to create the amazingly complicated reaction called a sneeze.

Good health is nothing to sneeze at, so trying one or two of these tonics when you have a fit of "Ha-choos."

APPLE CIDER VINEGAR

- For nighttime sneezing that sometimes comes along with a cold, lightly sprinkle apple cider vinegar on your cotton pillowcase before bedtime. Because apple cider vinegar may leave yellow stains on light fabrics, it's best to use an old pillowcase.

BAKING SODA & SALT

- Mix four cups of water, one-quarter teaspoon of baking soda, and two teaspoons of salt. Using a bulb syringe, quickly squeeze the mixture into your nasal passages for relief.

HONEY

- Eating a tablespoon of local honey daily is a swell way to relieve sneezing and its associated hay-fever symptoms.

LEMON

- Treat sneezing by heating an eight-ounce glass of water and add to it the juice of half a lemon. Mix well and drink.

SALT

- Boil a cup of water. When it cools a bit, but is still warm, add a teaspoon of salt into two tablespoons of the water. Using a clean eyedropper, place two or three drops of the salt solution into each nostril.

SNORING

Snoring from A to ZZZZZ.

Earsplitting and never-ending, snoring may sometimes bother your sleep-partner. Whether it's earth shattering or not, it can disturb an entire household. Truth-be-told, most folks snore at one time or another. It occurs when your breath flows past the relaxed tissues in your esophagus, making the flesh tremble and creating the throaty and annoying sounds.

Rest assured, dropping a few pounds, limiting your booze before bedtime, or catching your "Z's" by sleeping on your side may help. If not, try some of the following to let the rest of your household get some rest:

APPLE CIDER VINEGAR & HONEY

- Mix one teaspoon of honey and a tablespoon of apple cider vinegar with eight-ounces of warm water for an anti-snoring, pre-bedtime cocktail.

HONEY

- Letting a teaspoon of honey melt in your mouth every night before bed should minimize your snoring.

OLIVE OIL

- Sip some olive oil before bed to lubricate the throat muscles. This can sometimes stop you (or your partner) from snoring.

SALT

- Salt may actually cause snoring...so avoid it if you can.

SORE GUMS

If you don't take care of your mouth—good guess—your gums are going to be sore. Make good oral hygiene a regular part of your daily personal care by brushing your teeth a number of times each day for at least two minutes (as long as it takes to sing "Twinkle, Twinkle Little Star" a couple of times—in your head, of course) followed by flossing at least one time each day. Both will toughen your gums and keep them clean.

If your gums are sore, eat up these suggestions to help your healing:

APPLE CIDER VINEGAR

- To ease the discomfort of sore gums, make a mouthwash of one teaspoon of apple cider vinegar added to an eight ounce glass of water. Gargle and swish, and then rinse well with water.

BAKING SODA

- Occasionally brushing your teeth with baking soda will help to heal your sore gums.

HONEY

- Add three tablespoons of honey into an eight-ounce glass of water and mix well. Gargle with this mixture two or three times each day for best results.

LEMON

- Rinsing your mouth with the juice of one lemon added to an eight-ounce glass of water will eliminate the bacteria that create sore gums.

SALT

- To speed healing to your sore gums, mix one tablespoon of salt into an eight-ounce glass of warm water, swish it around, and spit out.

SORE THROAT

If you feel like you've just swallowed glass, and the accompanying scratchiness is making you bonkers, good guess is that you've got yourself a sore throat. A common sore throat burns, feels tight and really dry, and sometimes also hurts when you swallow. It's often the first red flag that you're catching a cold or having a reaction to pollen or dust. Your sore throat may also be caused by snoring, hollering, screaming, and even yodeling. Make your own alternatives to "cut-throat" commercial products:

APPLE CIDER VINEGAR & HONEY

- Combine ¼ cup apple cider vinegar and ¼ cup honey, and take one tablespoon every four hours or as needed.

BAKING SODA

- Add a half-teaspoon of baking soda to a glass of warm water and gargle with this mixture every thirty minutes. Spit and then rinse with plain water.

LEMON & SALT

- Add the juice of a lemon and one teaspoon salt to eight ounces of warm water. Gargle three times a day for a minute, spit, and rinse with pure water.

SPLINTERS (See Cuts and Wounds)

SPRAINS

A man with a wrench can put a new twist on sprains.

A sprain is an injury to your elastic-like bands—or ligaments—that attach your bones and hold your joints into place.

Ankle and knee sprains happen most often. They swell fast and hurt like the dickens. Luckily, most minor sprains can be treated at home. The following remedies should give you a leg up on relief:

APPLE CIDER VINEGAR

- Within the first forty-eight hours of getting a sprain, speed the healing by soaking a towel with apple cider vinegar, wrapping it around ice cubes, and securing it with a rubber band. Place the iced towel gently on the sprained area, leave it on for twenty minutes, remove it for twenty minutes, put it back on for twenty minutes; off for twenty minutes…on for twenty…. Repeat as needed. Because apple cider vinegar may stain light fabrics, it's best to use old or darker colored towels for this remedy.

OLIVE OIL

- Soon after the injury, gently massage the area with a teaspoon of olive oil.

STIFF NECK

A stiff neck occurs when the muscles in your neck and shoulders become tight and inflexible. In the worst-case scenario, the pain can be so severe that you can't move your head at all. Thankfully, most are entirely treatable at home.

So, if you're stiff with a pain in your neck (or even a working stiff who's a pain in the neck), consider trying these suggestions to ease your distress:

APPLE CIDER VINEGAR

- For a stiff neck, soak a towel with apple cider vinegar and warm it in the microwave. Be sure that the towel is not burning hot. Wrap the towel around the sore area, and leave it on for an hour. Repeat if the pain is not gone. Because apple cider vinegar may stain light fabrics, it's best to use old or darker colored towels for this remedy.

LEMON

- To get relief from a stiff neck, rub your neck with fresh lemon juice.

OLIVE OIL

- Warm a few teaspoons of olive oil and rub it into your aching neck.

CAUTION: *Don't confuse meningitis with sore neck muscles. A medical professional should examine anyone under the age of twenty-one years old with a stiff neck or anyone with both a fever and stiff neck.*

STIFFNESS

Stiffness can come from decades of wear and tear on your muscles and joints and can show up as a knee twinge, smarting feet, and maybe even throbbing ankles.

Don't be inflexible. Relieve joint pain with the following remedies:

APPLE CIDER VINEGAR

- When your muscles are feeling sore and stiff, add apple cider vinegar to your diet.

BAKING SODA

- Relax in a hot baking-soda bath by adding ¾ cup of baking soda into a warm tub of water to relax your stiff muscles.

HONEY & LEMON

- For stiffness, mix two teaspoons of lemon juice and a teaspoon of honey into an eight-ounce glass of warm water and drink it twice a day.

OLIVE OIL

- Massage stiff areas with warmed olive oil to provide relaxation.

SALT

- Apply a paper bag filled with warmed salt to relieve muscle stiffness.

STINGS & BITES, INSECT (See Insect Stings & Bites)

STOMACHACHE

Abdominal pain can be nothing more than an accumulation of gas or bloating and—in most instances—is nothing to get worried about. And because, since time immemorial, everyone has had a stomachache at one time or another, there are plenty of quick and simple homespun ways to treat it.

Here are a few stomachache remedies to keep under your belt.

APPLE CIDER VINEGAR

- Drink one tablespoon of apple cider vinegar and—within minutes—your stomachache will begin to fade:

BAKING SODA

- The classic stomachache remedy contains ½ teaspoon of baking soda added to about four ounces of warm water. Drink it straight down and wait for the belch.

HONEY

- Try eating ¼ teaspoon of honey before each meal to help prevent you from getting stomachaches.

CAUTION: *A physician should evaluate persistent abdominal pain.*

STOMACH, UPSET (See Indigestion)

STRESS

When you're reacting quickly and effectively while under stressful conditions, that's what's called "performing well under pressure." But when your stress center is sent into overdrive, that's when you'll start to see problems. Your system overreacts, and in turn, so do you—that's called "burn-out." It might not feel great, but stress is a normal reaction, as is the way your body copes with it.

To calm yourself during or after a stressful situation, consider these hassle-free alternatives:

APPLE CIDER VINEGAR

- To remedy the physical effects that often accompany stress, take a tablespoon of apple cider vinegar before each meal.

BAKING SODA

- Although stress hasn't been linked directly to heartburn, it's been known to lead to it. Dissolve a teaspoon of baking soda into eight ounces of warm water and toss it back for quick relief.

HONEY

- Take one teaspoonful of honey in eight ounces of warm water to get immediate relief from stress.

OLIVE OIL

- A massage with the tiniest amount of olive oil can give fast and easy relief from stress.

STRETCH MARKS

Crimson or pink sunken lines on your belly, boobs, upper arms, thighs, or butt are an everyday discovery to most pregnant women, and even men and women who have gained and then lost weight will spot stretch marks on their skin. Stretch marks are those superficial "dazzling" (but undesired) streaks on your skin that become paler over time.

Even though treatment can reduce their appearance, it won't be a stretch to try the following:

BAKING SODA

- Depending on the severity of your stretch marks, exfoliating with a paste of baking soda and water may be helpful to remove layers of dead skin.

OLIVE OIL

- Massage olive oil into your stretch marks to assist in their disappearance.

SALT AND OLIVE OIL

- Pour ¼ cup salt into a container and completely cover with olive oil. Stir and then gently massage the affected area and exfoliate your stretch marks away. Repeat daily until you're satisfied with the results. After each massage, shower and towel dry.

STUFFY NOSE

The term "stuffy nose" is frequently used to describe the oo-and-goo blocking the flow of air in your nose, whereas "runny nose" refers to the faucet of stuff filling your tissue or covering your sleeve. Together they describe what your nose is up to while you're experiencing the common cold or an allergic reaction.

If your nose is stuffy, don't block it when it comes to trying the following:

APPLE CIDER VINEGAR

- To relieve a stuffy nose, bring to a low boil ½ cup of apple cider vinegar added to ½ cup of water and breathe in the steam.

BAKING SODA & SALT

- Combine ¼ teaspoon of baking soda and ½ teaspoon of salt to eight ounces of water. Use an eyedropper to dole out the solution into your nostrils whenever you need relief.

LEMON

- Mix the juice of half of a lemon added to eight ounces of warm water and drink up to find relief from a stuffy nose.

SUNBURN

Prevention is the best remedy...especially when it comes to avoiding sunburn. Too much contact with the sun is damaging, so take precaution by using a sunscreen that's right for you. In the event that you still manage to get a sunburn, try one of these bright ideas:

APPLE CIDER VINEGAR

- For small areas of sunburned skin, apply apple cider vinegar to your skin with a cotton ball. For one of those real scorchers, prepare an apple cider vinegar-soaked towel as a cooling compress for larger areas to relieve the pain. Because apple cider vinegar may stain light fabrics, it's best to use old or darker colored towels for this remedy.

BAKING SODA

- Add ½ cup baking soda to a tepid bath and soak. Instead of drying your sunburned skin with a towel, let it air dry. Baking soda cools and will also help your skin retain its moisture.

HONEY

- Honey is a useful treatment for sunburn. Lightly apply it to your sunburned skin and cover with a dressing.

LEMON

- Mix the juice of three lemons into two cups of cold water and sponge this mixture onto your sunburn. The lemon will cool the burn, act as a disinfectant, and will promote healing of your skin.

CAUTION: *If you experience chills, fever, get blisters, or a rash, you may have sun poisoning. See your physician. Also, don't ever cover sunburn that is blistered or open with an ointment, oil, salve, or butter, for it will make the area susceptible to infection.*

S

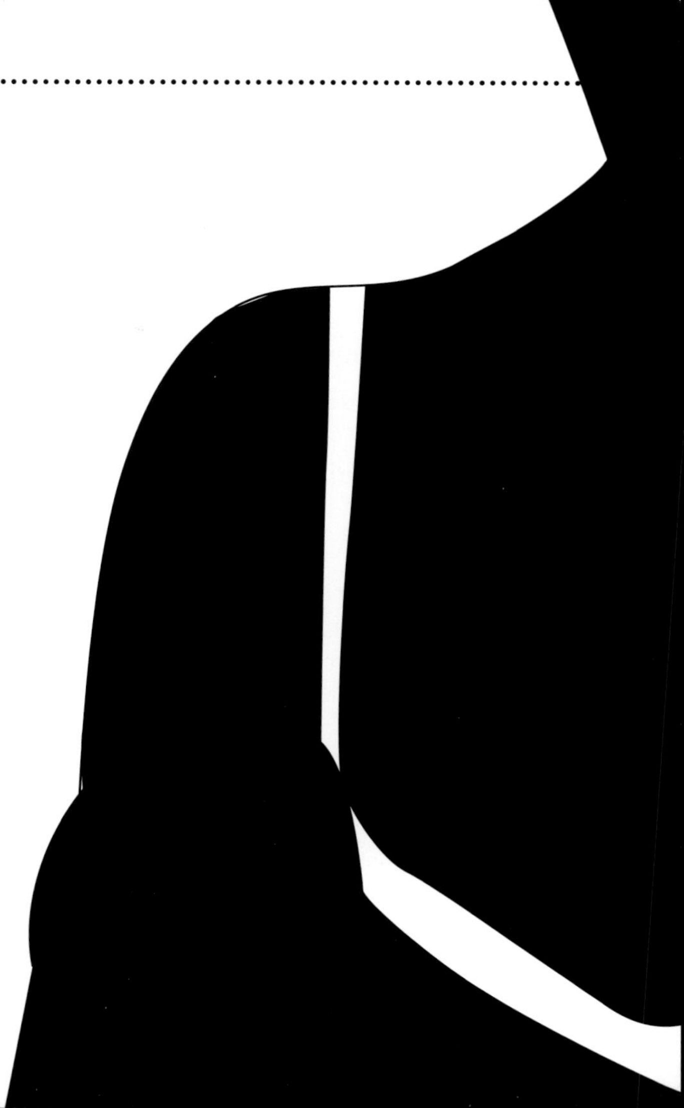

SWELLING

Caused by the build-up of fluid in your skin and other body parts, swelling commonly occurs to folks who have been standing or walking a lot and occurs most frequently when it's warm. Whether it's a lot of puffiness or just a little, you'll find the following remedies swell:

APPLE CIDER VINEGAR

- For minor swelling, create a mixture of half apple cider vinegar and half chilly water and soak a rag in it. After wringing, wrap the rag around the affected area. Leave it in place for about an hour—the longer you leave it, the better the results.

HONEY

- A light smear of honey helps reduce swelling.

CAUTION: *Generalized swelling is a common sign in severely ill people. Please consult a doctor.*

TOOTHACHE

Cavities are the root of most toothaches.

The primary cause of toothaches for kids and adults is tooth decay. Germs that inhabit your mouth live on the food that you eat. Producing a gummy plaque that adheres to your teeth, their acids eat through the tooth enamel. Proper daily cleaning often deters decay, so remember to brush after meals and floss daily.

Sensitive to sweets, cold, and hot, cavities can be painful and should be treated by your dentist. While you're waiting for your next appointment, sink your teeth into these remedies:

APPLE CIDER VINEGAR

- For a toothache, place a cotton ball soaked with room-temperature apple cider vinegar onto your affected tooth. This will relieve the pain of your toothache until you can see your dentist. After the pain has subsided, rinse your mouth with water.

BAKING SODA

- Gargle with two tablespoons of baking soda dissolved into an eight-ounce glass of warm water. Follow by swishing it around your mouth for forty-five seconds. Spit out the gargle and then repeat until all of the wash is gone. This will briefly minimize your pain until you can see your dentist.

HONEY

- Rubbing a dab of honey on your aching tooth can be effective on tooth pain. This will briefly reduce your pain until you can see your dentist. Make certain you rinse afterward.

LEMON

- Place a wedge of lemon onto your affected tooth to bring temporary relief from the pain of a toothache. Afterwards, rinse with warm water.

SALT

- One teaspoon of salt in an eight-ounce glass of warm water creates an effective saline swish 'n' spit that works best at the onset of a toothache. And yes…rinse.

U

UPSET STOMACH (See Indigestion)

URINARY TRACT INFECTION

A germ that begins in your urinary system can become a urinary tract infection, affecting your urinary system and especially your private parts and pieces. While women have them more often than men, they can be painful and exasperating to anyone.

Treating a urinary tract infection with antibiotics is nothing out of the ordinary, and in many cases is the necessary course of action. But the best medicine is prevention, and you can take steps to reduce your odds of getting a urinary tract infection in the first place. Use some of these hints to make your bladder gladder:

APPLE CIDER VINEGAR & HONEY

- Avoid urinary tract infections by mixing two teaspoons of apple cider vinegar and one teaspoon of honey to an eight ounce glass of warm water. Stir and drink it down once a day.

BAKING SODA

- Drink eight ounces of water with ½ teaspoon of baking soda to treat yourself at the first hint of urinary tract discomfort. If you already have a urinary tract infection, this remedy should help reduce any pain.

LEMON

- To help clear up a urinary tract infection, drink a potion of 50/50 cup of lemon juice and water each morning.

CAUTION: *If you are pregnant or have diabetes, you should be evaluated further by a medical professional because of the risk of miscarriage in the former and kidney infection in the latter.*

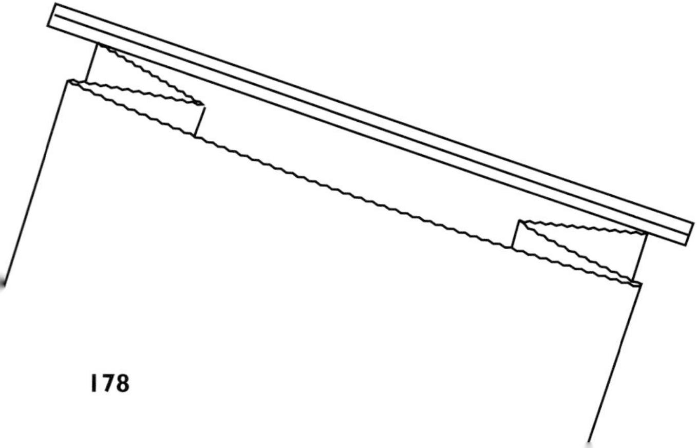

VOMITING

Vomiting is never a gag.

Adults and kids will puke from overeating, overimbibing alcohol, food poisoning, indigestion, motion sicknesses, pain, pregnancy, stress, viruses, and even out-of-control odors. If not a sign of a more serious illness, it's normal to hurl once in a while. And if you are heaving, drink plenty of fluids to decrease your odds of becoming dehydrated.

So if you feel the urge to upchuck, barf, spew, or retch, follow your gut feelings and choose one of the following effective treatments to settle your stomach:

APPLE CIDER VINEGAR

- To treat vomiting, stir one tablespoon of apple cider vinegar and one tablespoon of honey in an eight ounce glass of water and drink before bed.

BAKING SODA, HONEY & SALT

- To treat the dehydration that often accompanies vomiting, combine two tablespoons of honey, ¼ teaspoon of salt and ¼ teaspoon of baking soda with four cups of water. Stir well and sip throughout the day.

LEMON

- The smell of freshly cut lemons is extremely helpful when treating your nausea and vomiting.

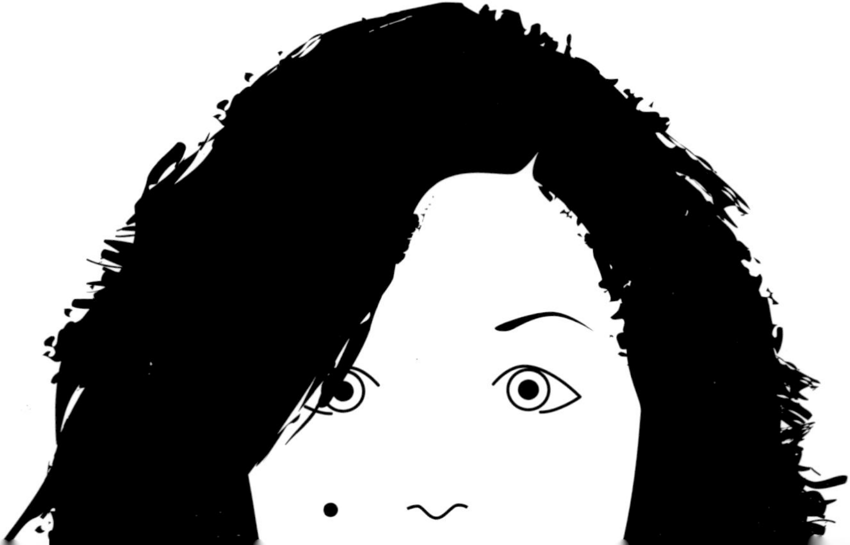

WARTS

Warts have a funny way of growing on you.

We've all had warts somewhere on our bodies and, other than being a bother, for the most part they're harmless. Therefore, it's not always crucial that they be removed because, without treatment, they often disappear by themselves anyway.

But if you feel a need to assist in their exit strategy, flesh out your situation and then mull over the following preparations:

APPLE CIDER VINEGAR

- Soak your wart in warm water for twenty minutes; dry thoroughly; apply full strength apple cider vinegar with a cotton ball and leave on for ten minutes; wash off with tepid water and dry with a clean towel. Repeat as needed until the wart goes away.

BAKING SODA

- Rub the wart three times daily with a solution of 50/50 baking soda and water. Allow the area to air dry.

HONEY

- Apply honey to a wart and cover with a bandage. Continue to apply honey and a fresh bandage each morning and night until the wart disappears.

LEMON

- Rub fresh whole strength lemon juice gently into your warts. Repeat two or three times daily until your warts disappear. Don't wash the lemon juice off; just allow it to air dry.

SALT

- Moisten salt and apply it to your wart. Follow by covering it securely with a bandage. Continue this process until the wart disappears.

WEIGHT LOSS

Eat less and burn more—you know the drill. While losing weight, try simple things like eating more fruit and vegetables, consuming less fat, and getting off of your butt and moving. In an attempt to swing your scale into the opposite direction, here's some food for thought:

APPLE CIDER VINEGAR

- Drink two teaspoons of apple cider vinegar mixed into an eight-ounce glass of water three times a day to assist in your weight loss plans.

HONEY & LEMON

- Consume the juice of ½ lemon and a teaspoon of honey mixed into an eight-ounce glass of warm water each morning to help curb your cravings.

WINDBURN

Windburn is when your skin, exposed to the elements, gets dried, chapped, burned, and appears red and swollen. Not to be confused with sunburn, windburn is less damaging to your skin.

If you've thrown caution (and your skin) to the wind, consider the following for relief to your sensitive skin:

APPLE CIDER VINEGAR & OLIVE OIL

- Mix equal portions of apple cider vinegar and olive oil and apply a small amount onto exposed skin to protect it from windburn.

BAKING SODA

- Cool the effects of windburn irritation by applying a paste of three parts baking soda and one part water directly to your unhappy hide.

LEMON

- Mix the juice of three lemons into two cups of cold water and sponge onto your wind-burned skin. The lemon will cool the burn, act as a disinfectant, and will provide care to your crust.

WOUNDS & CUTS, MINOR

Cuts, scrapes, scratches and punctures are a result of an accident or injury. Minor wounds usually aren't life threatening, but even nicks and abrasions require TLC.

To sidestep contamination and aid healing:

- Use pressure and a clean cloth to end bleeding
- Tidy the wound with soap and water
- Use an antibiotic ointment to avoid infection
- Bandage the boo-boo
- Check for any changes
- Get a tetanus shot if you've not had one in the past five years

If your standard solutions aren't making the cut, think about using these:

APPLE CIDER VINEGAR

- Since apple cider vinegar helps blood clot, a weak solution of apple cider vinegar and water can be applied to minor wounds or cuts.

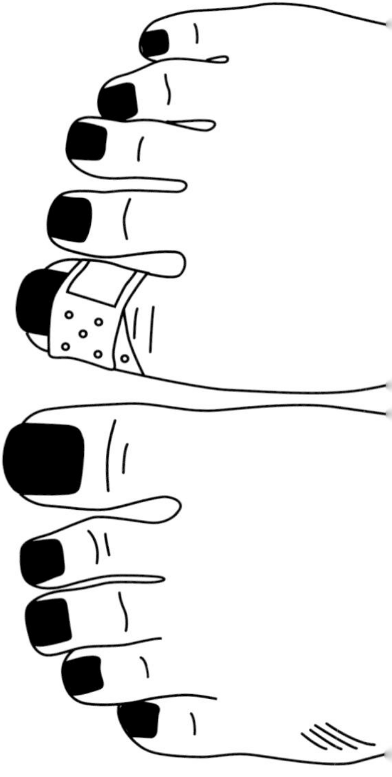

HONEY

- Dressing a minor wound or cut with honey provides a physical barrier to infections. Clean the site, dab it on and then cover with a sterile bandage.

LEMON

- The disinfectant qualities of lemon juice when applied to a freshly cleaned, minor wound or cut will aid in healing. Once done, affix a sterile dressing.

OLIVE OIL

- Protect minor wounds and cuts from infection with an application of warm olive oil. Clean your wound, lightly dribble some olive oil onto the area, and then cover with a sterile bandage.

SALT

- Make a paste of salt and water and apply it to your minor wound or cut. You'll probably scream bloody murder, but if you have an infection you'll see it disappear right before your eyes.

CAUTION: *Serious and infected wounds require professional medical attention.*

WRINKLES

Growing old means wrinkles—and if you've been baking in the sun or have been sucking on cigarettes, you'll probably have more of them sooner. The fat in your skin disappears, your skin starts to sag, and those wicked wrinkles materialize.

Everyone gets wrinkles because it's part of aging. However, applying the following preparations at any age can be a smooth move.

APPLE CIDER VINEGAR

- Take a cotton ball, dip it into apple cider vinegar, and then apply it directly to your wrinkles. This remedy won't diminish your wrinkles, but it will bring a divine, rosy glow to your face.

BAKING SODA & HONEY

- Mix equal portions of baking soda and honey and apply this elixir directly to your wrinkles. Leave it on overnight and delight in the difference in the morning.

LEMON & OLIVE OIL

- Remedy your wrinkles by applying lemon juice directly to your age lines and leaving it there for two hours. Rinse with warm water and then massage the area with the tiniest bit of olive oil.

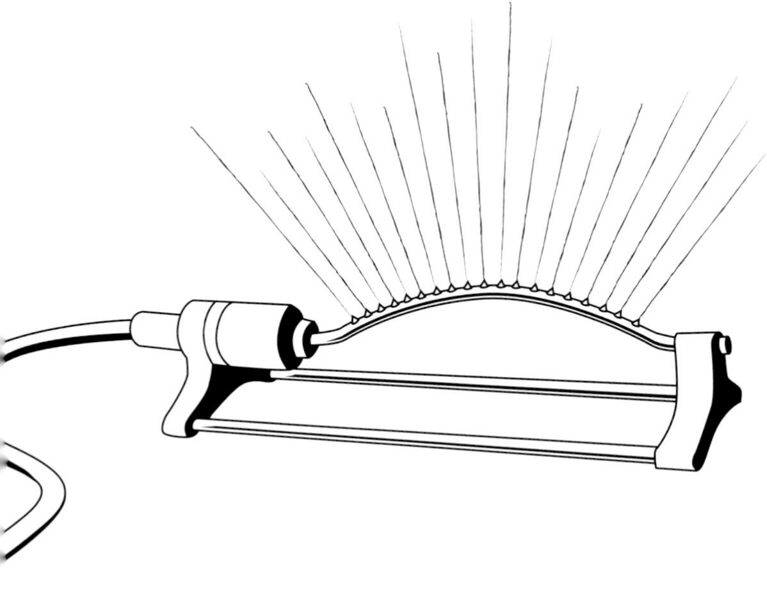

YEAST INFECTION

Completely common, yeast is a fungus that—more often than not—survives in the vagina in minuscule numbers. When a vaginal yeast infection occurs, it signifies that yeast cells are overdeveloping in your vagina. Although they're always aggravating, yeast infections aren't dangerous. Periodically use these simple treatments when yours are acting up:

APPLE CIDER VINEGAR & SALT

- Add half a cup of vinegar and half a cup of salt to a warm bath and soak for at least fifteen minutes. Dry thoroughly.

BAKING SODA

- Add ½ cup of baking soda to a lukewarm bath. Soak for fifteen to twenty minutes twice daily until your symptoms have cleared up. Towel dry.

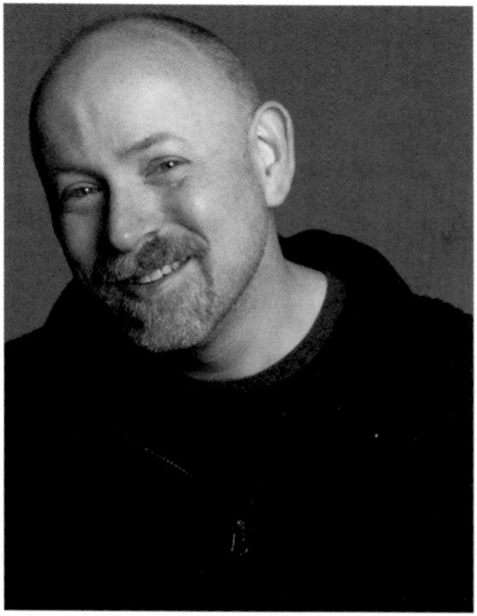

Photo: David Herrenbruck

Author Michael De Jong is an environmentalist and eco-activist living in the New York area with his partner, Richard, their dog, Jack, and three goldfish, Gill, Jill and Bill.

He blogs for The Huffington Post, The Daily Green and Intent, as well as for his own site, www.MyKindofClean.com.

He is the author of *Clean: The Humble Art of Zen-Cleansing* and *Clean Body: The Humble Art of Zen-Cleansing Yourself. Clean Cures: The Humble Art of Zen-Curing Yourself* is the third book in his My Kind of Clean™ series for Sterling Publishing.

De Jong donates a portion of the royalties from his My Kind of Clean™ series to the OneCleanWorld Foundation, his not-for-profit charity that supports eco- and sustainability projects in the U.S. and abroad with grants, technical assistance and/or micro-financing.

For more information about the foundation, visit www.OneCleanWorld.org.
To contact Michael De Jong, email him at Michael@MyKindofClean.com.